The Hero Of the Story

Reclaiming Your Life After a Multiple Sclerosis

Diagnosis

Meagan L. Freeman, MSN, FNP-BC

Published 2015 by Pearl Glow Books, LLC

For inquiries contact: pearlglowbooks@gmail.com

Printed in Charleston, South Carolina, USA

ISBN: 978-0-69240-559-8

Library of Congress Control Number 2015937317

Preface

This book was born after a period of time writing my blog, *Multiple Sclerosis, Motherhood, and Other Traumatic Experiences.* It has been a labor of love, one that got me out of bed in the morning for quite some time. I searched for a way to continue to heal and help others after my career began to slow due to MS. I hope that every reader will find the experiences and advice contained within helpful and positive, and through my own life experience I hope to continue to heal others.

I was diagnosed with relapsing remitting multiple sclerosis in 2009, in the midst of my education to become a Family Nurse Practitioner. I had been an emergency department registered nurse for 8 years when I was diagnosed, and had 6 children at home. At this point, I was faced with a life changing decision. Did I continue with my education despite the diagnosis, or quit?

This book is divided into sections focused on a specific illness related topic, and each section is followed by a journal prompt. These are journal prompts designed to help readers work through their own experiences with these situations, and to write down feelings, thoughts, and ideas. I have found through countless interviews with fellow patients that most chronically ill patients experience a similar process of grief and acceptance after diagnosis, and you may find that you experienced these same thoughts and emotions.

I have always found journaling to be one of the most therapeutic, effective techniques for venting trapped emotions, gathering thoughts, and keeping a log of ideas for future use. Please feel free to stop and think about each topic, and write down some notes for yourself for later. If you want to truly achieve something by reading this book, you should take a moment to write something at each journal point. Some of these notes may even be helpful to show to healthcare providers or family members and friends to read.

I hope that every reader, whether a patient, caregiver, or loved one will appreciate this information and find it helpful. Stay strong! You may just find yourself becoming a hero.

Foreword

"Don't ever miss the opportunity to look at your patient's brain." This is one of the innumerable axioms that spin in the minds of physicians every day as they care for their patients. My earliest recollection of hearing this was during my Neurology rotation as an Emergency Medicine resident. Dr. Kaufman, professor and chair of Michigan State University's department of Neurology and Ophthalmology, recited this in his lectures and during hospital rounds. He was referring to the performance of a thorough ophthalmologic exam and taking the time to evaluate the retina, which is essentially brain tissue, for clues to systemic disease. Optic neuritis, a common initial presentation for MS, where patients present with sudden loss of vision, is one such disease.

One of best ways to "look" at the entire brain is with an MRI. As a residency trained, board certified Emergency Physician I had seen my share of MRIs during my first 13 years of full time practice. The MRI I was looking at on August 24, 2009 was of a patient's entire brain and spinal cord. It was full of what I have come to call "even-I-can" lesions, because even I, as a non-radiologist, non-neurologist, could see them. The only difference this time, it was my wife's MRI and the lesions were classic for MS.

Emergency physicians are trained to "think worst first" when evaluating and treating patients in the hopes of never missing a catastrophic disease process. This mantra works well in the clinical setting, but not so in one's personal life. Having seen many MS patients at their worst, I could only envision "the worst" possible future for my wife. One filled with walkers to wheelchairs, diapers to catheters, and ultimately disability to death.

In the Emergency Department, making the diagnosis is both the challenge and the endpoint. As I have learned, however, the real work comes later. It's the patients, their families and their personal physicians who have to find a way to accept, cope, manage and live with their new "normal".

In her book, Meagan takes you through her personal journey from health care provider to patient and back. Importantly, she focuses on the unseen impacts chronic illnesses like hers can have on one's identity, outlook and goals. While sharing her story, she encourages her readers to journal aspects of their own experiences, and in the process, create a framework for the personal restoration of self. Anytime a healthcare professional can provide a therapy devoid of drugs and surgeries, they have done their patients the greatest service, and fulfilled their role as advocate. By that measure, Meagan has accomplished this laudable goal.

Dr. Wayne Freeman
Emergency Physician
Santa Rosa, California

The Hero of the Story

For Bette, the MS fighters, and others
yet to be diagnosed.

Contents

PART ONE: DIAGNOSIS

1

A Moment Replayed a Thousand Times

"All great changes are preceded by chaos."
-Deepak Chopra

Sometimes, memories of my pre-diagnosis life haunt me, like ghosts in the foggy distance, dreaming of a life that was destined not to be. I imagined myself as a dancer, gymnast, long distance runner – so many things. I loved them all, longed to keep them in my life, but had to let them go. Oh, how I miss that carefree former self! The one who thought I was untouchable and life was easy. We design a life for ourselves, but that's not how it works, is it? Life constantly challenges us to make the most of what we have – not what we wish we had. And sometimes, in our darkest hours, we find out how strong we truly are.

The music played from my car stereo as I drove, *Hotel California* blaring from the speakers, moving along Highway 101 toward my home. The familiar landscape of that stretch of road passed by in a blur, and I tried not to think too much about this day. I glanced uneasily into my rearview mirror. There was my mother Susan's gray Subaru, directly behind me. She had that unmistakable look of concern on her face – the tight mouth and knitted brow as worry lined her forehead beneath her bangs. Anxious, yet trying to hide it for my sake, as she'd done with so many problems in the thirty-four years she'd raised me as her only child.

The last thing on Earth I wanted to do was to cause her any more anxiety and stress. "God let this not be the day that I break my mother's heart," I thought to myself. Suddenly, a sound interrupted *Hotel California*, not a sound I wanted to hear. It was the ringtone on my iphone, that annoying ringtone you always hear; I meant to change it, but never got around to doing it. I glanced over at the screen, and the hospital phone number stared back at me. I felt my skin grow prickly, and the nausea started to rise. No, I thought. No no no!. I didn't want to answer that call. *I didn't want to know.*

A few weeks earlier, my husband Wayne and I took the kids to San Francisco. It was one of those perfect, sunny, summer California days, the sky swept clean by ocean breezes, white sails cutting through the whitecaps of San Francisco Bay. As we crossed the Golden Gate, bikers and joggers were out in droves. Couples held hands, pushed baby strollers, paused to take in the awesome views.

When we saw Pier 39 across the bay, our excitement grew. The kids love Pier 39, with its herds of barking sea lions, live music, fun attractions, and lots of good things to eat. Wayne and I had six kids, and all of them were with us that day: Shawn, 12, Dylan, 10, Braeden, 8, Audrey, 7, Lindsay, 2, and Katy, 11 months. Everyone was healthy and happy, and no one was arguing for a change. If it weren't for the nagging itching I felt on the back of my head, it would have been a perfect day.

By the time we reached Golden Gate Park and saw the Frisbees flying, I was scratching constantly. Since Wayne is an ER doctor, I asked him about it, but it didn't strike him as serious. After working together for five years in the ER, we learned to trust each other's judgment about medical issues. We figured he could check my scalp when we got home. The irritation calmed down and eventually stopped, and I pretty much forgot about it.

Wayne and I were fairly newly married. We had the "Doctor and Nurse fall in love in the ER," made-for-TV movie type of love story. We were both married previously, and went through difficult divorces at the same time. There is something about working in that stressful environment that brings people together. We had so much in common, and meeting him felt like coming *home*.

We were married in the summer of 2007, just after the birth of our oldest daughter, Lindsay. We planned the entire event in one day, and everything just fell miraculously into place. We were married in a beautiful preserve for ancient redwood trees in Northern California called Armstrong Woods. There is a small theater within the park, a beautiful, quiet, magical place, like something out of a fairytale. Sunlight cascaded through the historic lofty branches of these trees above us that had seen so much history pass below them. We said our vows there, with the sun just rising above the forest, our friends and family looking on. I walked slowly down the aisle of shredded redwood bark, breathing in the smells of a fresh, natural morning. It was a day of love and happiness, ending with our arrival at a rustic Lake Tahoe cabin for the week. A honeymoon with five children is not entirely private or romantic, but I cannot remember ever feeling as relaxed and carefree as I did on that day in July.

After returning from our honeymoon, life continued as it always had. Although we thought nothing of it, I recall coworkers asking, "How can you possibly work with your husband? Don't you get into arguments?" It wasn't a problem for us. We drove to work together, worked long shifts, and drove home together afterward. Looking back, it was one of the most content periods of my life.

Around Christmas of 2007 I had been nauseated and feeling a bit fatigued, and it just did not seem normal for me; I slept constantly, and just felt like something was wrong. Then, I missed my period. I thought to myself, "There is no way in hell I can possibly be pregnant again. This cannot be happening." We already had 5 children to care for! I raced to the store to buy a pregnancy test, and hurried home to take it. I saw that pink line start to develop slowly, and I felt lightheaded. I remember walking slowly toward Wayne, who was busily changing a diaper on our 10 month old. I stood in silence and stared at him, and he eventually looked up from the diaper disaster he was wrangling. "WHAT?" He asked the question out of pure concern, given the look on my face. I replied, "Oh my God. I am pregnant *again.*" Obviously, we were both medical professionals, and knew how to prevent another pregnancy. I suppose we both knew the possibility was there, but maybe we secretly wanted just one last baby. It's one thing to imagine a child, but entirely another when you actually see a positive pregnancy test.

Our sixth child Katy was born in August of 2008, after a stressful, high-risk pregnancy. I developed hypertension, as I had with my other four children. I had been on bed rest for the last month, and Katy had to be induced one month early. I recall that my legs would occasionally become numb and itchy during this pregnancy, but who had time to consider it? I ignored the intermittent numbness and carried on with my busy life. In general, I felt very well, much better than I ever did when I wasn't pregnant. Katy did quite well under the circumstances, and ended up a strong 6 pounds, 15 ounces. She was a smiling, happy, dark-haired girl. I was grateful to deliver a healthy baby after the dangerous complications I had experienced.

As if we didn't have enough going on at home, I decided to return to school in 2009 to pursue my Bachelor of Science in Nursing. Wayne's achievements as a physician were a major source of inspiration for me, and I wanted to be a provider like he was. I wanted to be independent, rather than just carrying out orders all day long as an RN. My goal was to obtain a Master of Science in Nursing and Family Nurse Practitioner licensure. I wanted to feel that achievement, and Wayne was a constant, unwavering source of motivation. "Education is never a waste of time," he would tell me. He encouraged me, listened, and showed complete confidence in my abilities.

Near the end of my Bachelor's program, in August of 2009, I began to feel a tingling sensation on my right upper chest. It was a particularly hot summer day, and Katy was having her first birthday party. We had company over to the house, and an enormous cake for Katy. She tore into it, frosting covering her tiny mouth. I held her on my lap as she opened her gifts, and when she leaned back against my chest it became obvious that I couldn't feel anything on the right side. The small area of numbness on my right ribcage proceeded to expand, growing larger and larger each day. We have all experienced numbness of some kind, maybe after a dental procedure or when a foot falls asleep. This was like no numbness I had ever experienced. It was completely dead. My torso felt as though it was not a part of my body at all, and when I touched it, I may as well have been touching someone else. There was no sensation whatsoever from my clavicle to my hip on the right side.

Wayne did not tell me how concerned he was at the time, attempting to protect me from unnecessary stress. He later said that he was almost certain I had a neurological illness of some kind, but he didn't want to worry me excessively. I knew this numbness wasn't normal, but I carried on, went to work, dropped children at school and made dinners. In a way, I suppose I was in denial. This was my classic coping technique, just pushing everything from my mind and pretending all was well. Healthy? Not really. But it's tough to change those personality traits. This was my way of dealing with fear.

After a day or two of this dense numbness, Wayne and I looked at each other. There could be no more denial; we needed to have this evaluated. Wayne spoke to a neurologist friend who ordered an MRI and some lab work. We were aware of my family history; with my grandmother having multiple sclerosis. MS was in our minds, but I just could not believe that was the explanation. I refused to accept that as a possibility, I made assumptions that I was special, untouchable, *nothing bad will ever happen to me.*

The "BANG-BANG-BANG" and shrieking siren noises blasted my ears despite the earplugs I had been given. The Velcro-laden straight jacket hugged my arms securely, preventing me from moving in any direction. The brace held my head, preventing me from turning side to side. The ceiling of the tiny tube hovered inches from my face, making me feel like some sort of futuristic space traveler, hurling through the universe. The feeling of being inside a closed MRI tube is terrifying to many people. Because of the claustrophobic nature of this test, many choose to be sedated during the 90-minute procedure. I chose to go ahead without sedation, and I was regretting that choice! What incredible thoughts ran through my brain during those 90 minutes, an entire life review. Was I going to die? What was going on in my brain? How would my children survive without a mother? How could this actually be happening?

On my way out after having my MRI, I stopped by the ER, our place of work, our home away from home, filled not just with colleagues, but friends. Being a patient in my own ER was one of the strangest experiences of my life. My mind felt confused, foggy, baffled. I should be *here working*. I quickly cut the hospital band from my arm, embarrassed.

I had no desire to be a patient. Wayne was working that day, and he knew I was having my MRI. He wasn't at his desk. He was busy, in a patient's room, a man who had a cardiac arrest. A room full of docs and nurses were working to save him. The CPR continued, and I could hear Wayne calling out orders for more medications. I stood, staring ahead at the crowded room, the curtain half open. I felt alone at that moment. Lost, like a stranger in my own workplace. I chose not to wait or interrupt him. I left him a small, handwritten note on his computer as I left, "Just had my brain MRI. Headed home. Talk to you soon, love you," and then I left.

Here I was, on that familiar freeway, before the days of "hands free only" cell phone use; that ring of my phone sitting on the car seat next to me, will echo forever in my memory. I recall the spot on the road, and every time I pass it I remember vividly what happened that day. Behind me on the road, my mom followed. She had witnessed first hand the slow decline of her own mother, who suffered from an incredibly progressive and destructive case of multiple sclerosis, and had died from complications in her fifties. As the oldest of seven children, she was forced to take over the load of household responsibilities at around age 12. My mother's family members were survivors of the ugly, destructive nature of this illness, one that took their mother away at a young age. MS was the monster in the nightmare, the beast lurking in the dark shadows of the closet.

The phone rang again, and then again. The hospital number on the screen told me what was coming. I heard that screaming in my head: *"No, no! I don't want to know!"*

I finally hit the talk button. It was my friend Hilary, another emergency physician at the hospital. Her voice was quavering.

"Wayne wanted me to call you, he is too upset to talk," Hilary said. "He's in the back room, trying to deal with this. He couldn't even listen as I made this call."

Even over the phone, I could hear a very strange tone in her voice, one I had never heard from her before.

"I'm so sorry, Meagan. Your MRI is abnormal. You need to get back to the ER right away."

"What is it?" I asked, managing only a whisper. Then louder, frantic, "The MRI! Tell me!"

She said in a low voice, "Our working diagnosis is multiple sclerosis."

My heart sunk, I forced myself to take a breath. There was no exit for another mile, and I didn't think about pulling over on the side of the freeway. I was in a robotic state. I kept driving, half of my mind was listening to the voice on the phone, and half was lost. Like Alice falling through the rabbit hole, time and everything around me seemed distorted and unrecognizable. At age 34, that moment was the death of my youthful, naïve self.

I pulled my car from the freeway at the nearest exit, my mother following behind, completely unaware of what had transpired. We pulled into the parking lot of a local coffee shop, and I threw open my car door, tears streaming from my eyes and stood there, staring at my mother. "I have it, Mom. I have MS." My mother hugged me in the middle of that parking lot, crying along with me. "We will get through this, Meagan. We will figure this out somehow," she said, somewhat unconvincingly. My mother's thoughts must have placed her right back to her childhood, watching her own mother slowly waste away due to MS. Now, her only child, the one she had protected for so many years, was the next victim. I could only imagine the pain she felt, how ironic and cruel the universe could be, and my immediate thoughts were of her. I apologized to her, knowing how much this hurt, "I am so sorry Mom. I am so sorry...."

We returned to the ER, where I would now be the patient. Nurses are not used to being patients, and this just felt so wrong! We walked slowly into the hospital, holding onto each other for support. We were ushered into one of the rooms, and I was wrapped in warm blankets while tears streamed down our faces. Coworkers passed my room, looking at me with sad, sympathetic eyes, not the sort of looks I was used to receiving. I smiled back, pretending all was just fine. I did not want sympathy.

I began to have the second and third MRIs needed to fully evaluate a potential MS diagnosis. The MRI technician made his way to my side, holding a large syringe with a white substance within. I recall seeing him walking deliberately toward me with a stone faced appearance, letting no emotion show. He said in a monotone voice, "It's time to inject the contrast," and began to access my IV port. I looked down at the IV in my arm, and reality truly sunk in. The contrast entered my vein, with the intent of "highlighting" the damaged areas of my brain and spinal cord on the MRI images. That contrast was on its way, heading toward the potential lesions, and it would soon tell me what I needed to know.

The hum and whirring of the MRI continued. Other than the blasting, loud noises, the only other experience I recall was thinking, "I am really sick. There is something seriously wrong with me." I heard the MRI technician whisper quietly to the nurse: "She is one of the ER doctor's wives. This is not a normal MRI." They may have thought they were being quiet, but I heard them.

After the exam was finally complete, I was told that I had MS. It was definite, and there was no longer any question about what had caused my numbness. There was a sense of relief at that point, and I felt grateful that I did not have something far worse, such as a tumor. Leaving the MRI trailer, I was transported by wheelchair through that summer day, along the parking lot I once used to wheel countless patients out to their cars. I was supposed to be the one pushing the chair. Feeling like I was in a nightmare, I was sent to a hospital room on the third floor, and greeted by the first of many nurses who cared for me. Those nurses were incredible, empathetic, attentive, sweet, and so helpful. I wish I could have told them what a difference they made for me in those early hours, when my entire life and identity were being put to the most frightening test. *Who was I now?*

Quitting school was something that I thought about almost immediately, and over and over for months. I tried to ignore those demotivating voices in my head, the ones that said, *"You should just stop now. What is the point? Take the easy road, forget it."* I was halfway through my Bachelor's program, should I quit? I was just going to end up in a wheelchair. Bedridden. Nonverbal. Just like my grandmother. What was the use of finishing school? What was the use of doing ANYTHING now? My future now would consist only of being a "sick" person, with doctor's appointments, imaging, blood work, medications, and progressive decline. Images of my grandmother raced through my mind.

The 3-night hospital stay was like an out of body experience. My husband could not stay with me during the evenings and nights, because someone needed to be home with the children. I was alone, in the dark, with a hardened hospital mattress to sleep on, and I was fed the classic "microwave dinners" hospitals always serve. I could not recall the last time I had so much time to myself. Unfortunately, this was not the ideal way to get that precious time alone. The nurses changed shifts, checking on me once or twice. My vital signs were taken, and I was in no pain. I hate to complain about much typically, so I sat in silence most of the time. I didn't dare press the call light for fear of irritating my nursing colleagues. Anytime someone peeked into the door and asked how I was doing, I put on my classic fake smile and said something like "I am doing just fine, thank you!" How could I possibly explain how I was actually feeling? How could I describe the devastation, the loss, the grief, and the confusion? How would I go on like this forever? There would never be another day in my life when I was not *sick*.

The experience of having three days of high dose intravenous steroid infusions is something that cannot be explained. Steroids induce pseudo *insanity*. The mind races, anxiety grips you, and you become incredibly paranoid. The symptoms of an MS flare do not typically resolve immediately just because steroids are used. The symptoms drag on for weeks or even months, despite treatment. So, I was left with dense numbness, extreme fear and anxiety, steroid side effects, and a stunned mind. Of course, once I returned home, life would demand that I carry on, my children would need me, my job needed me, and schoolwork loomed in front of me.

After three days of steroid infusions, instructions in interferon self-injection techniques, long discussions with my neurologist, and the acquisition of a new identity, I was discharged home. I recall the neurologist saying that my case had a particularly poor prognosis because of the numerous lesions seen on my spinal cord. Many patients present with only brain lesions, but I had many throughout my brain, spinal cord, and a case of transverse myelitis. I was almost certainly destined for rapid decline. "We tend to observe family member's progression as a gauge for your possible progression," my neurologist told us. The only other family member with MS was my grandmother, who was severely disabled by the time she was 45. Things did not sound good for me.

Journal 1: Diagnosis:

Do you remember your diagnosis day? What do you recall? What were your feelings, your fears, and your experiences? What did you find most helpful in that moment?

2

Suffering Disappears, Love Remains

"Not all of us can do great things. But we can do small things with great love." -Mother Teresa

When my diagnosis occurred, the assumption my mother and I had was that I would end up just like my grandmother. The words "multiple sclerosis," were so terrifying because of the images they conjured in our memories. Every chronic illness comes with an image, usually a negative one, of decline and degeneration. My grandmother was a beautiful, intelligent, energetic woman who was reduced to a shell of her former self after decades battling MS. This woman was a military veteran, a strong individual who never allowed anyone or anything to dictate to her. She lived in a time of male dominance and misogyny, yet found a way to show courage and strength instead. Tragically, the one thing that seemed to have complete control in the end was MS. Bette became bedridden in her late 40s, and eventually died from MS complications at 55. This was the fate that we believed I was facing, and this was the cause of our panic and fear at that moment. MS was a beast in the family closet, a nightmarish fiend that took our loved ones from us.

As a child of 5 or 6, I have vivid memories of visiting the home of my grandparents. We spent many holidays there, the home where my mother and her 6 siblings grew up. My grandfather, Stan, was the breadwinner, and my grandmother Bette slowly declined while trying to raise her 7 children. She had been diagnosed with Multiple Sclerosis in the 1950s, when there were no treatments available. She was basically told to "get in bed and stay there." Faith, love, and hope were the keys to their success, and my grandparents were a living example of heroism and true love despite devastating life circumstances. We've all seen those movies with an unbelievable story, where love conquers all, however this one is true.

When I feel weak, I think of them. When I feel overwhelmed with my lot in life, I think of them. When I want to give up, cursing the universe for the bad hand I was dealt, I think of them. When I question whether truly unconditional love exists, all I need to do is recall this life story and look at their pictures. You see, what matters at the end is our life story, our legacy, the story that will be told to future generations. Each of us is slowly writing a story that will be told someday, and it is incredibly important that we write one that we will feel proud of.

My grandparent's story began on a Southern California beach in the 1940s, just after World War II began. It was love at first sight, according to my grandparents. My grandfather describes my grandmother as "the most beautiful girl he had ever seen." They sat that day on the beach, my grandmother in a yellow bathing suit under an umbrella, sipping beers together. They were immediately drawn to one another, a fated meeting. Life was never going to be easy for them, but they would not have it any other way. From that moment on, they hung onto each other through it all, never giving up on this commitment. They both joined the military during the war, my grandmother serving as a WAC, my grandfather in the Army Air Corps. Soon after, they married and started a large family, eventually having 3 girls and 4 boys. My mother was the oldest girl, and took on a great deal of responsibility for her younger siblings.

This beautiful love story began to take a turn. That beautiful image, that perfect wedding day, the meeting on the beach, the love that brought these two together. This is the foundation of a relationship that would truly stand the test of time, and the test of multiple sclerosis. Sometimes, difficulties bring out the best in people. Sometimes it takes struggle to find out *who we really are*, and what we are truly capable of. Sometimes, it takes a crisis to find out how much we are loved by our family and friends, and how far love can carry us. My grandparents were about to experience that struggle first hand.

My grandmother began to experience new neurological symptoms, new emotional instability, and eventually, seizures. The health history of my grandmother is somewhat unclear, because this was occurring in the 1950s, before MRI, before a solid understanding of multiple sclerosis. After years of symptoms and hospitalizations, my grandmother was eventually diagnosed with MS. At this time, the disease was poorly understood, no treatments whatsoever were available, and the advice was to lie down, don't exercise, and essentially just wait to die. Can you imagine? As we now know, this is just about the worst possible advice for an MS patient.

A wheelchair made its appearance when my grandmother was in her 40s, and eventually she needed daily nursing care and was bedridden. My memories of my grandmother consist of days spent visiting her on her bed, watching TV, and carefully observing as she was fed her liquid meals through a straw. Bette would smile at me, with beautiful, kind eyes as I sat with her. I knew she sensed we were all there, but she could not verbalize much. Her bed was warm, cozy, and comfortable when I was five. I loved to grab onto the bedrail, and swing my legs beneath the bed, and my cousins joined me. We laughed, sang, and talked with our grandma, who did not respond in the traditional verbal way, but rather with smiles like no other.

When faced with the option to move Bette to a nursing home, my grandfather refused. He insisted that she stay in the home, with the family, no matter how difficult it was. His seven children would not grow up without their mother present in the home, even if her physical decline was upsetting. Here is the beautiful part of the story: My grandfather decorated a beautiful, sunny bedroom for his wife. He hired a caregiver, Elsie, who was a wonderful part of the family, present every day to care for the seven children and Bette while he worked. He included his wife in every celebration and family event, and he must have been physically and mentally exhausted. He worked full time, served as husband, father of seven, caregiver, and breadwinner. Most are overwhelmed parenting one or two children, let alone seven.

The family continued to grow, with myself and many other grandchildren making an appearance. Family Christmases, weddings, and other celebrations always included my grandmother. I recall my grandfather lovingly styling her hair for a family gathering, knowing he would be ready to take many pictures. Hundreds of photographs were taken over the course of their lives together, and we are fortunate to have this documentation now. The love between my grandparents could be felt strongly if you were near them, and for many years, the love grew and the care continued. Eventually, however, Bette lost her battle with MS.

My grandfather lived on for another 15 years, gardening, visiting with many grandchildren, and enjoying holidays with the family. He would always say that he was going to see his wife again someday. He got a very specific expression on his face when he talked about Bette. His smile changed, and his eyes would drift off skyward, as if he were having an actual conversation with her. He never doubted that he would see her again when he passed away, and he was waiting patiently for that day. The strength of the human spirit is incredible, isn't it? The ability of a human being to sustain the daily grind, work, children, marriage, illness, and even death is remarkable. The depth of our strength cannot truly be known until we face challenges like MS. We must undergo many changes in life, adapt, overcome, and go on.

On their grave is the quote "Suffering Disappears, Love Remains." When you think about it, isn't that the truth? Our suffering isn't permanent. It isn't forever. Every single detail of our lives is temporary, and that is the key to learning to truly be "in the moment." We must begin to understand that nothing is ours to own, but only to borrow for a period of time. However, do you know what *is* forever? *Love.* With my own diagnosis, I have seen my grandparent's story as a source of inspiration. There is no "I can't." I can and I will. This story demonstrates that MS will not stand in the way of the love of family and friends. MS may actually have a role in promoting love, caring, healing, and devotion among family members.

Multiple sclerosis was my family's enemy. It was something to be terrified of, something to dread and despise. In such a large family, everyone waited to see who would be next. Would any of my grandmother's 20+ descendants be the next victim? As a child, I recall spending hours reading books and raising money for the National MS Society "Read-a-Thon," and my mother encouraged me to help the cause. It was our family's cause, and the disease had impacted us so severely. Raising money for MS research gave us hope and made us feel powerful in a powerless situation. At 34, I became the latest victim of the family enemy.

Like my grandmother, I had a very large family with 6 children. The similarities were incredible, and like my grandfather, my own husband became my supporter and caregiver. He was my rock, and I could not have been more fortunate. Having MS gave me such a new perspective on life. The little things that used to seem important are meaningless. Now I realized that love, family, friends and fun are what make life worth living. When you feel that your time to enjoy life is limited, you begin to actually live. The truth is, none of us are getting out of this alive. We all have a limited time in this realm, so why waste a moment of it? I am grateful for MS at times, as strange as that sounds. I am grateful for the perspective and gratitude it has given me. If it weren't for this illness, I may still be sweating the small stuff. I may still be blindly wandering through life, unaware that my time is precious.

So in the end, the family enemy may well have been the best friend anyone could have, as strange as that sounds. A friend who has shown me what is truly important in life. When you feel that life has handed you a lousy deal, keep in mind: You are strong and capable. Your strength comes from a place deep within, and you won't believe how strong you can be when you have to. Lean on those around you when you need to.

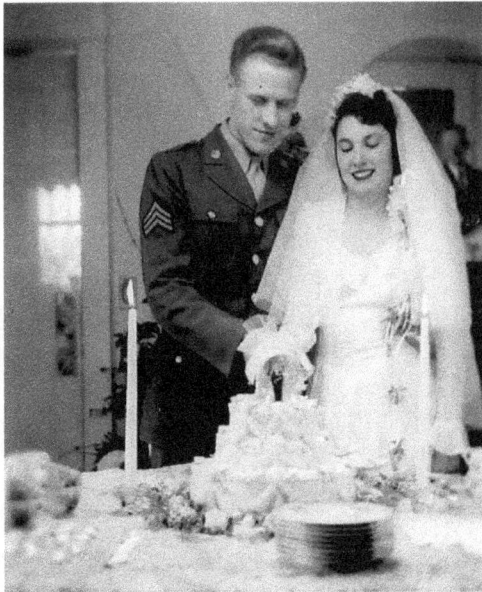

My grandparents on their wedding day, 1945

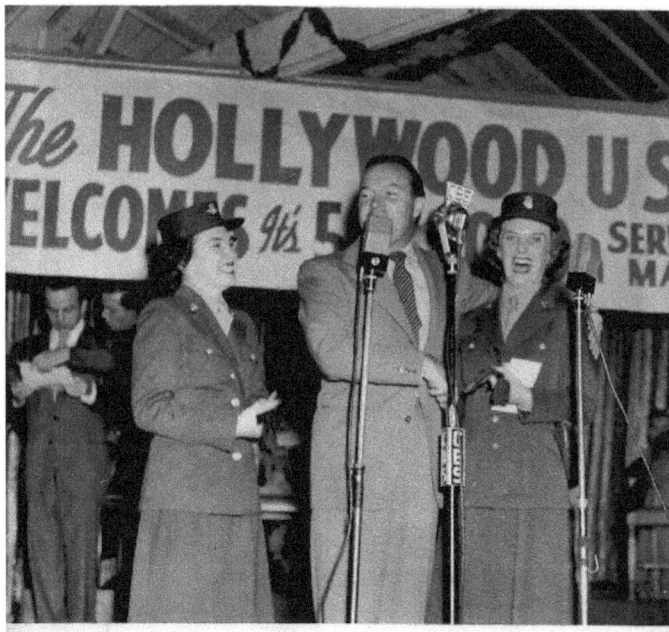

Bette with her best friend and Bob Hope at the USO

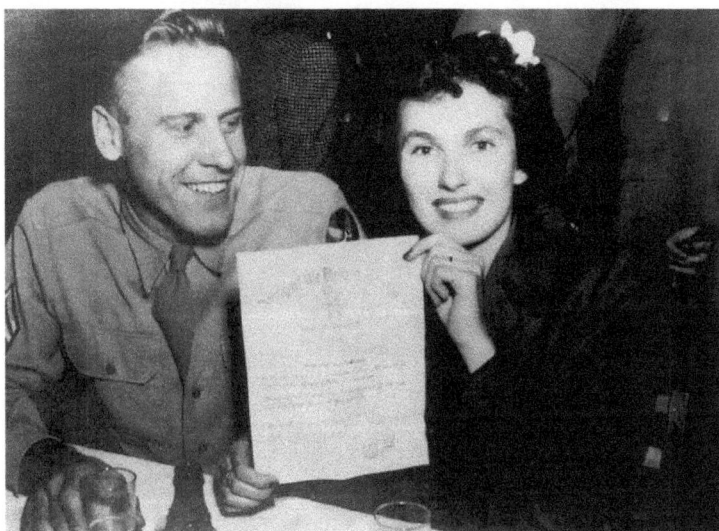

My grandparents, receiving Bette's honorable discharge, 1945

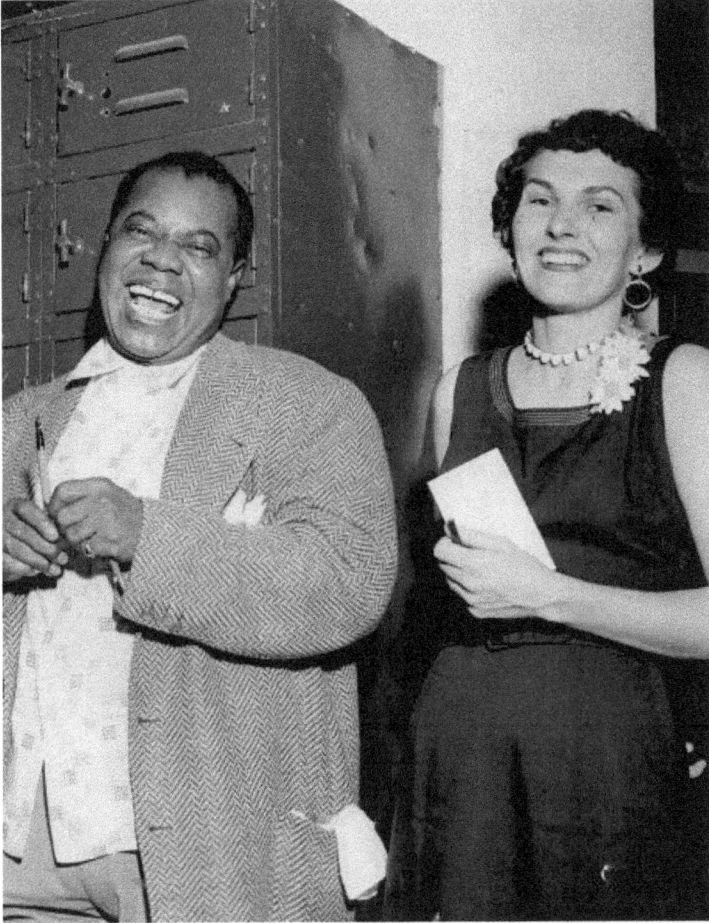

My grandmother with Louis Armstrong, 1960s

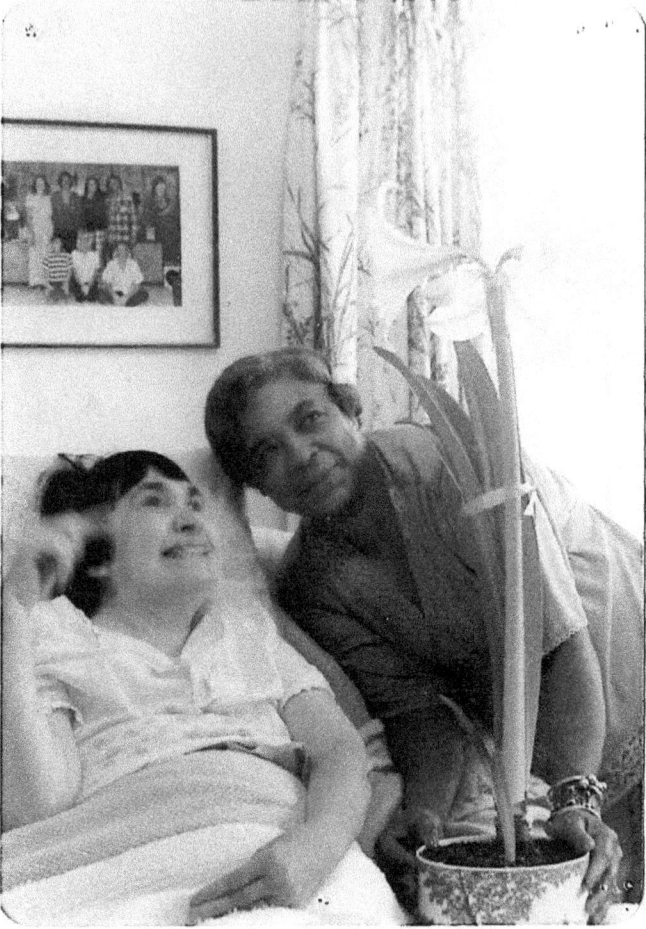

My grandmother with her caregiver, Elsie

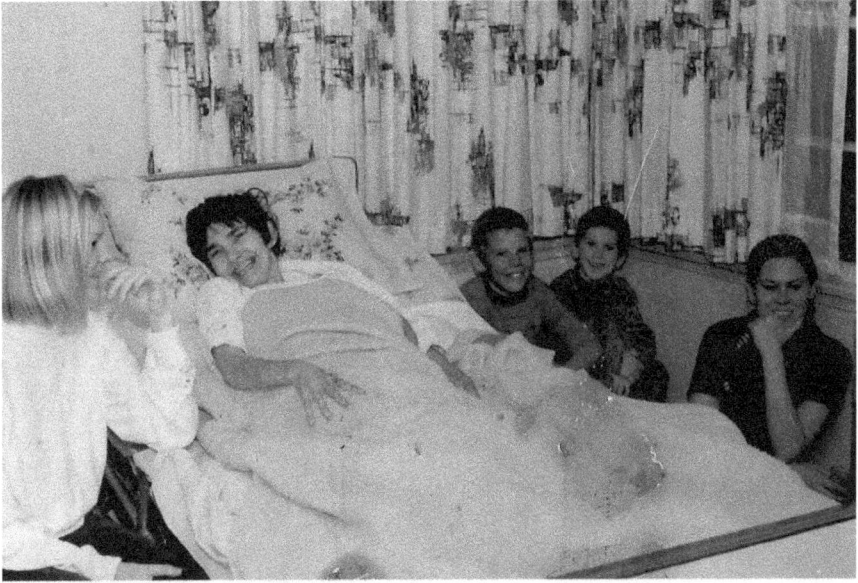

My grandmother, mother, aunt and uncles, 1960s

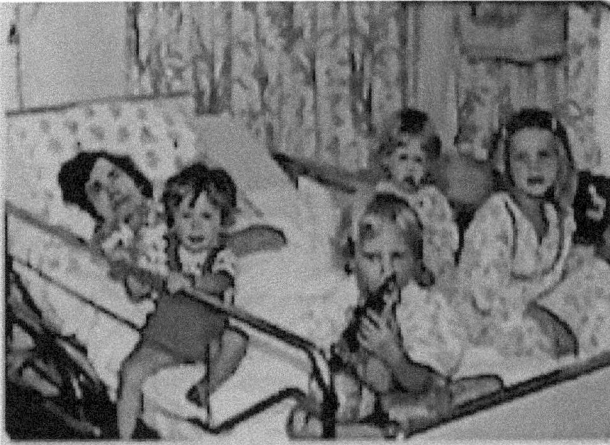

My cousins and I, on Grandma Bette's bed, 1976. Though a bit grainy, it is the only photo I have of my Grandma and I together.

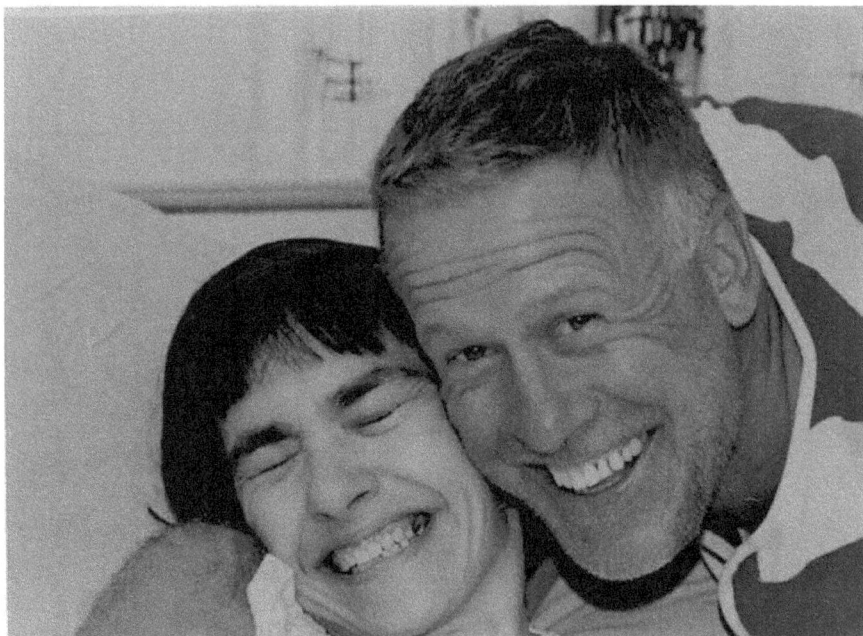

My grandparents, near the end of Bette's battle with MS. Still madly in love...

Journal 2: Inspirational People:

Can you think of any particularly inspirational people in your life? Do you have a hero? Someone who guides you and inspires you to be a better human being? Have you ever thought that you might be someone's hero someday?

3

I Don't Have Time
For Multiple Sclerosis!

"Denial helps us to pace our feelings of grief. There is a grace in denial. It is nature's way of letting in only as much as we can handle." -Elisabeth Kubler-Ross

As a mother of six, I had very little time for anything. Simply using the bathroom took planning and precise timing, so I clearly did not have time for the diagnosis of multiple sclerosis. Who would? I had kids at home who needed laundry done, dinner needing to be made, and my ten-page essay on nursing theory due the next day! How was this even possible? Why would I be the only descendant of my grandmother to be diagnosed with MS? This was so unfair, so unjust. Why me? I asked myself this question dozens of times over the last five years. *Why me?*

Upon discharge from the hospital, it was time to go home and return to normal life. It is important to understand that people do not simply assimilate a new

34

identity overnight. This process takes a great deal of time, patience, and perseverance. Was I supposed to just step back into my role, take care of my children, keep my house clean, get back to work, be a wife and mother, and pretend as if life would just continue? In addition, I had a full time Bachelor's program to complete, in which I had invested hundreds of hours and thousands of dollars. I had no choice in my mind, and I had to keep marching on. What would be my final story, that I was diagnosed and promptly quit everything? I gave up? I refused to try? This could not be my story, I would not allow it.

I dragged myself to clinical hours on days I would rather have stayed home. I sat through lectures, fighting the urge to sleep due to fatigue. The years of daily battles to attend clinical and classroom training rolled on, and learning to put other's needs before my own was a strange irony. My IV infusions, the steroids, the blood tests, the MRIs and the neurological evaluations became a blur. The line between patient and healer was unclear, and the role I played on any given day could change dramatically based on my physical condition. I was stalked by demotivating voices in my head, and they were contemptuous, cruel and discouraging. I did not understand where these voices came from, but only that they caused me to seriously question every move I made. It was as if this diagnosis, this label of "MS" had caused me to view myself in a totally different way. My former self-confidence had dried up and withered away, now replaced with an utterly self-conscious, self-destructive image.

While the diagnosis is a physical one that can take years to evolve, the emotional toll becomes immediately apparent. I never knew a day in my life when I questioned myself intellectually or academically. Those were my strengths, and I could always depend on my brain to get me through any situation. Now, I imagined my brain under attack, lesions, scars, and inflammation. This formerly dependable mind had become completely unpredictable, and it was now my weak point, not my strength. Processing this complete change in self-image is extremely difficult for newly diagnosed patients, and it is difficult to describe to those who have not experienced it first hand.

Somehow, I ignored these internal demotivating creatures that wanted me to stop. *"What are you thinking? Why are you even trying this? Give UP,"* they would whisper. I learned to push them aside. Late nights studying massive medical texts, strain of the eyes, and heavy backpacks hauled across a seemingly endless campus became my life for years. I doubted my ability to complete this program because of this diagnosis. This was a very realistic fear, for according to everything I read, what I had was *incurable, degenerative, and disabling.*

When I returned to normal life, the new identity slowly seeped in. One thing that shocked me about being a patient was how isolating it was. I lived with seven other people, a cat and a dog and a bearded dragon lizard. In a house filled with chaos, clamor, shrieking, screaming, fighting, barking, meowing, slamming of doors, blaring of music, din of TV, and mayhem of computer gaming, how was it even possible that I would feel so alone?

I felt that my experience with illness was unique among the people I knew and cared about. On bad days, I found myself yelling at my loved ones "You don't understand! You can't possibly know what I feel like! You don't have THIS DISEASE." I always felt terribly afterward, seeing the looks of sadness on their faces. They wanted to understand, they tried, but how could they? With a rare illness, affecting only one in one thousand in the US, I knew no one else currently living with the disease. At these moments I never missed my grandmother more. What words of wisdom would she have for me?

Kids just do not seem to understand when you are ill. They see you as a parent, strong and capable, no matter what. Mom is my hero! How can she be too ill to get me more ice cream? The transition from diagnosis day to normal life was a bumpy, emotional road. Over and over again, I found myself feeling that no one cared about my diagnosis. The problem was, my children still needed all of the things they needed before MS. They needed meals, clothing, baths, and rides to school. My husband could not take time off work, and he still needed to be there during all sorts of insane hours, working in the ER. This left me with much time alone, pondering my new identity. I found myself becoming resentful as I continued writing term papers, mothering, keeping house and working as a nurse. I could not rationalize that I had become a patient with an incurable disease. This was my denial phase, the time when I pretended to be healthy, though I was not. I pretended to be strong and happy when I was, in fact, terrified of every moment of my life. This fear and anxiety may have been the fuel that drove me on during this period of my life. Fighting was the only option I had.

I carried on, and cared for my emergency department patients as if nothing had changed. I pushed the gurneys, inserted the IVs, gave the medications, performed the chest compressions, and all the while my mind was somewhere else entirely. "I hate you, you bitch!" The psych patient bellowed from the locked psych room, after I walked out. Once again, I had refused to give the patient the dangerous, unnecessary narcotic medications she was demanding. "Meagan, your patient needs you," yelled another nurse. I ran to the room to find my patient with a colostomy standing in the middle of the room, stool leaking from the ostomy site. As he stood, a river of liquid feces flooded the doorway. For the uninitiated, I will tell you that the smell is indescribably noxious. Grabbing a bucket, I helped the elderly man to the restroom, and consoled him as he apologized. I cleaned him up, and got him back to bed. As I knelt on the floor mopping up the mess, I felt so bad for him, but all the while I was thinking, "Why am I still doing this? I don't know how much time I have left to be a physically functional person. I need to find something else."

I returned home that evening to my children, and all were predictably needy. They were always so clingy after I worked a long shift. I bathed them, fed them, and changed a few diapers, feeling like I was going to collapse from exhaustion at the end of the day. I knew I needed to find a career that required my cognitive skills more than my physical ones. I needed to plan, and I needed to do it quickly; I could feel my body beginning to fail me, and time was running short.

In the spring of 2010, I completed my Bachelor of Science in Nursing. This accomplishment was extra sweet, because I knew how close I came to abandoning the process altogether. I immediately began my application process for the Masters program at Sonoma State University. I knew this was a competitive process, and that only 40 spots existed in each new class. I would be competing with the best of the best. My disease made no difference in the acceptance process, and no one would give me special consideration simply because of MS. This was the first time I realized that I could not allow my disabilities to be an excuse to give up, to work less, or play the victim. I had no choice but to compete, to achieve, and to demonstrate that MS was not a barrier to success.

In May 2010, I received my acceptance letter in the mail, and I felt all of the chains I had been dragging around for 18 months drop away. I felt a resurgence of my former self-confidence, that foundational piece of my identity that had been so forcibly ripped away, and I knew I could succeed. I held that letter in my hands, trembling with tears rolling down my face. This was a moment like no other, one I would never forget, and one I would return to whenever I needed a source of hope and inspiration. I would begin the program in August of 2010, and attend a full time graduate medical program. This would be my biggest challenge to date. Could I keep up? What if I was having a relapse, and could not attend class? I knew how strict these programs were, and I was worried, with good reason. I may have finally gotten in over my head with this endeavor.

Journal 3: Motivation?

What do find motivating? What drives you to get up and fight when your body is screaming at you to lie down and rest? What would you say to another patient experiencing demotivation and fatigue? Pretend you are coaching another patient, and write your own "pep talk"

4

Who Do I Blame For This?

"When one door of happiness closes, another opens; but often we look so long at the closed door that we do not see the one which has been opened for us."
-Helen Keller

On particularly difficult days, the world seemed to be gray and heavy, light was dim and my mood was bleak. Life refused to stop for me, however. I wanted it to, but it would not. It did not matter to the world that I was ill, and no one would pay my bills for me. I felt bitter, angry, and resentful toward healthy people at times, and I did not completely understand these feelings. I had no time to go on a worldwide tour and "find myself" somewhere on a lost island paradise. I had no time to relax, have a massage, and ponder life. Life just picked right back up where it stopped during my hospital stay, and I was displeased.

Not only was I coping with my regular life obligations, my children, my marriage, and my job; I was now struggling to bring my lifelong dream to fruition. Finally, I had been accepted to this graduate program, and life had handcuffed me with this horrific disease. I experienced days in the cold rain, parking a mile from my classroom. I had a numb, weakened left leg and a broken umbrella, stumbling over cracks in the sidewalk as the pellets of cold water struck me from head to toe. My bag felt like a tremendous anchor, dragging me down with the load of massive books. I questioned everything during these moments, including my seemingly ridiculous pursuit of higher education. Why was I never just satisfied with what I had? Why was I always attempting to pursue more? Where was this endless, dissatisfying journey going to lead? I assumed it would end in abject failure.

I felt that life had it out for me. I thought I was being victimized by the universe, and I had no idea why. I had worked my entire life to help others, to make the world a better place, and to heal the sick. Why would the universe have chosen me to endure this? *Why me?* I searched for someone to blame, and I came up empty handed. This got me thinking, why do we always need to find someone at fault for our negative circumstances? Why is this automatically our response?

Isn't it interesting how we, as human beings, always feel better when we can "assign blame" for a perceived insult? My observation is, many people do this, including myself, and it is probably a very bad habit to get into. The blame game will not leave you better off in the end, will it? If you can blame your problem, whatever it might be, on another person, you will still have your issue, won't you? How do we disconnect from this age-old habit as patients? With many chronic illnesses, we can potentially blame our genetics, our ethnic background, our geographical location, the environment, and possibly viruses. But still, in 2015, we have no solid evidence as to who or what is responsible for many chronic diseases. Would it matter?

Having a chronic illness is a great way to learn that you cannot always find someone at fault for your problems. I suppose the key is to stop blaming, and start *living in spite of it.* We can blame the "system" for our lack of disability benefits, our employer for our lack of health coverage, and our families and friends for not understanding the struggle we go through. We can blame our treating physicians for not diagnosing us quickly enough, not treating us appropriately, or not being sympathetic enough. We can blame society for not taking care of the disabled more appropriately (some countries do a better job of this than others.) However, in the end, even if some of these issues are spot-on, we are still left to live with this illness until a cure is found. We are challenged to not only survive, but to actually live our lives to the fullest extent possible.

Remember, you still have many contributions to make to the world, regardless of your physical condition. If you are having a difficult walking day, perhaps try to use your cognitive skills a bit more. On days I felt weak, I tended to become the best at writing and expressing my feelings. We need to find a purpose and passion, as simple as it might seem. Purpose is a very individual concept, and you must be in charge of figuring out your own, no one can do this for you.

Sinking into the depths of negativity is a dangerous trap for patients, and we must be aware of this slippery slope. It is so tempting, especially on bad symptom days or during relapses, to turn to the dark side. We often start to feel alone, isolated, and angry at the universe in general. We need to stop this train of thought before it completely derails us, and recognize the first signs of negative thought processes. Feeling misunderstood, judged, and isolated is a common experience for many MS patients. A repeating theme among patients I have encountered is the frustration they feel at the lack of understanding of the illness, and the lack of support. I find that most people who hear the words "multiple sclerosis" have one of two reactions: "The disease is horrific, disabling, fatal, and basically a death sentence", *or* "what's the big deal? Isn't that just some minor little thing?" Both of these concepts are incorrect.

MS lies somewhere in the middle of those ideas, but the misconceptions come from lack of education. In addition, the wide variety of disease manifestations and rate of progression between patients causes great confusion. Often, I hear individuals describe someone they know with MS, and they apply those ideas to all patients. "My friend is doing just fine," or "my friend is bedridden," therefore, you must be experiencing the same thing. Either way, being judged is hurtful.

When we hear that MS is "no big deal," and we should be "doing fine," we feel dismissed, ignored, and belittled. Many of us have "invisible symptoms," things no one else can perceive, yet they cause much pain for us on a daily basis. Many have suffered dozens of disabling relapses, but have recovered and now appear fairly normal. To hear that it is "no big deal," discounts our experience, and our pain. When we hear MS is "basically a death sentence," we know this is incorrect. However, it is still hurtful, because it creates negative feelings, causes anxiety, and creates fear. We all know that we can still lead long, happy lives with this disease, but misunderstanding can still have an impact on us psychologically.

Once we receive our diagnosis, we have a responsibility. We should take on the challenge of educating our friends and family about our illness. We become the teachers, the educators, and we are responsible for ensuring that everyone we come in contact with will have an understanding of our illness. MS is still considered rare, with the prevalence being approximately 1 in 1000 in the US currently. By this statistic, we can see that we will all encounter someone in our lives who is "clueless" about our illness. We should see this as a clear obligation, to disseminate accurate information everywhere we go.

These prejudicial ideas are nothing but stereotypes, and we should do everything in our power to wipe out ignorance when it comes to our illness. Unfortunately, we may even encounter medical professionals who are not well educated when it comes to MS. Even in these situations, it is our obligation to try to educate.

Many health professionals do not specialize in Neurology, and have very little experience and training regarding MS. Don't hesitate to pass on information everywhere you go, and try to reference legitimate resources of information. If you find that anyone won't take your word for it, simply access a reliable site such as the Multiple Sclerosis Association of America (MSAA): http://www.mymsaa.org, or the National MS Society: http://www.nationalmssociety.org. Your credibility will increase when you reference other established sources of information.

Despite the fact that MS can have so many negative impacts on your life, you cannot allow it to get in the way of your hope and plans. Though it can be limiting and isolating, the challenge is to find a way to cope and look beyond. Don't write off tomorrow because today was not what you wanted it to be. Illness can also be the unlikeliest of teachers. Let me recount the lessons and "AHA! Moments" that MS has allowed me to learn:

1. Life is precious and fleeting, don't waste a moment.

2. The people who truly love you will always be there, no matter what your physical condition may be.

3. Your family and friends want you *present,* even if you are less than perfect.

4. Let go of your perfectionism, and accept what *is.*

5. Let go of the need to please others, it's an impossible task.

6. Learn to be grateful for the things you do have, and focus less on what you don't.

7. Learn to let go of your vanity, it is a waste of time and energy.

8. Accept more, control less.

9. Value your time in this life, rather than just watching the clock and counting the years.

10. You are much stronger than you ever imagined.

I am sure more items could be added to this list, but these are the ones that truly stand out in my memory. I have changed more since my diagnosis 5 years ago than I ever did in the 34 years before I was diagnosed. I have tried to become an individual who appreciates rather than envies, is thankful rather than needy and jealous. I am far from perfect, but I am making progress.

Challenges are opportunities in disguise, and you should try to see them that way. I know it is so much easier to give up, be angry, and hopeless. But it isn't the best mindset. Do whatever you can to avoid the temptation to sink into a depressive state, and instead turn yourself toward the positive. Chronic disease is horrible, destructive, and terrifying, but try to remember that things could be *SO MUCH WORSE.* This small statement is something I have repeated internally for the past 5 years on a very regular basis. Things could be worse. Things could be worse. Until I finally realize that they indeed could be.

I hope that you find these words uplifting and helpful. If so, try to give this advice to other patients you find who are feeling lost and hopeless. Helping others is one of life's greatest gifts. In the process of enriching one person's life, you will also find that you gain purpose from the experience. Giving to others serves a dual function; to assist someone in need, and to enrich the life of the individual providing the assistance. Giving to another human being shows the person in need that someone actually cares, and this alone might change a life. When I found myself turning inward and starting a "pity party," I strived to turn outward instead, and reach out to help another patient. It is certain that another patient could use your expertise.

When you are coping with your first year or so after diagnosis, you are going through a tremendous shift in thinking. Do not expect to feel inspired and positive at first. Sometimes, the first year is for learning, processing, and growing accustomed to your new diagnosis and identity. Do not give up hope. Trust me, there are thousands of us out there who are living full, wonderful lives despite illness, and you will be one of them! *Find your reason to try today.*

Journal 4: Blame:

Do you find yourself blaming others for your circumstances? How can you avoid that behavior in the future? Can you think of a positive spin to put on your challenges?

5

Acceptance

"Miracles come in moments. Be ready and willing"

-Wayne Dyer

As I was driving home from another morning of school drop-offs, something came over me. I could almost feel my Grandfather's presence in my car, encouraging me. I needed something to motivate me at that moment, and he was in my mind. This man was a hero during his life, and he was also a writer. I always had the "love of writing" gene, which I am sure was directly from him. The desire to write cannot be taught or learned, and it drives you until you release it onto the page. Would anyone care about what I had to say? Would anyone be interested in hearing my opinions or my life story? I suppose that was none of my business. What I needed to do was write my story, and let it be.

As I sat there I began to cry, yet I didn't understand why. Since I was a young child, I had the urge to live life in fast-forward, doing everything as quickly as possible, with urgency. I felt as though my life would not be long, and I needed to experience as much as possible in my allotted time on Earth. At times, this may have seemed like youthful stupidity to those observing my life choices, but in reality I wanted to experience life to the fullest.

Unfortunately, things do not always work out the way you want them to. Marriages end, friendships change, and sometimes, illnesses make decisions for you. Would I ever have the chance to swim on a beach in the Mediterranean? Would I see Europe the way I had always wanted? Would my children be embarrassed to be in public with me someday? Boy, my thoughts could sure get dark. Anxiety could take hold and pull me out of reality very quickly if I allowed it to. *Yet, writing could be the most therapeutic experience.*

No matter what challenge I was coping with, I found that if I sat down and poured those feelings onto paper, I was refreshed and renewed; it was much like traditional therapy with a counselor, except the paper was my therapist. The words were my medication, and the process of putting my thoughts and emotions into words was my cure.

I am a rather shy person, and some would say I am quiet and private. I had a few extremely close friends and family, but I keep my circle small. The interesting thing is, when I sat down to write, I had no trouble communicating and expressing my feelings. Words were my favorite form of expression. Whereas spoken words leave your mouth and cannot return, written words can be erased, changed, and edited after you have reviewed them.

When coping with a chronic illness like MS, expression of feelings is incredibly important. It is so easy to feel alone and without friends who understand. Journaling and writing is a great option for those who feel uncomfortable talking. "People who journal find a higher sense of self-awareness and are able to reduce anxiety and gain a sense of empowerment. Many people who struggle with deep emotional conflicts or traumas are unable to express their feelings in a verbal or physical way. Journaling allows a person the freedom of expression without fear of retaliation, frustration, or humiliation." (http://www.goodtherapy.org/journal-therapy.html#)

My journaling experience evolved over time, and my hope was that my writing would continue to help me express the feelings I had about each challenge with MS, parenting, and life in general. In addition, I hoped I might have the opportunity to continue to heal others through my writing.

In my practice as Family Nurse Practitioner, I encouraged my patients to journal when traditional therapy was not appealing to them. Some of my patients used writing as an adjunct to traditional therapy, and found it extremely beneficial. From feedback I received from my patients, my suspicions about the therapeutic effects of writing were confirmed. I would encourage anyone coping with illness, trauma, death, or simply life stress to try jotting down a few ideas onto paper. My rough days were improved when I spent time journaling, and this technique was one of the tools that got me through my years of higher education.

There were many days during my educational pursuit that could have spelled the end for me. The day I had my first episode of optic neuritis could have stopped me, I woke up with an extraordinarily painful left eye, dim and dark, refusing to focus. It was much like looking through a broken pair of sunglasses, smudged and dirty, but only on the left side. The day I woke with left foot drop could have stopped me, I had to drag my leg across the campus to reach my class, hoping that the hoards of youthful, carefree undergrads wouldn't stare. It was the first time I used my cane in a public place, purely out of necessity. Although I was self-conscious, it was a fear I quickly got over when faced with the option of not graduating. Just as journaling helped me cope emotionally, my cane was helping cope physically.

Many MS patients find that using assistive devices such as canes and walkers in public is an obstacle, purely because of vanity. Before my diagnosis, I never even noticed these objects as I made my way through a public place, other than to offer a sympathetic glance, or perhaps hold a door for someone who was struggling. After all, I was a career healthcare professional, used to seeing these things on a daily basis. These objects were part of my daily job, helping the elderly walk down the hallway with walkers, teaching patients how to use crutches and canes. They symbolized infirmity for me, a medical device, something that meant weakness, illness, and dependence. After diagnosis, these devices and what they symbolized took on an entirely different place in the forefront of my mind. In one year, I went from needing no devices to using a brace and occasionally, a cane. My brace looked like a robotic leg, and my children started calling it "mom's leg" because it sat upright in a shoe in the hallway. This step was an incredibly difficult one for me, although the devices themselves were very helpful. The physical effect was achieved, helping me to feel stronger and more balanced as I walked with my left foot drop. This was an amazing, light device that was easy to use, and invisible in long pants. I went from hobbling around my house to going out in public again and ambulating for a period of time. This was a huge deal! Why then, did I have such conflicting feelings about it?

It felt like coming out of the closet. Most of us are able to hide our diagnosis, at least for a while. That moment when you realize you can no longer cover up this illness is a tough one, and I was experiencing it fully. The stares are incredible, aren't they? I was used to getting "disapproving glances" for many years from strangers when I was out with my children, who inevitably act out in public. Those judgmental stares, when people seem to be thinking, "What kind of parent are you?" These new stares were different. Now I was the recipient of the sympathetic looks from strangers. Now I was the one getting doors held open for me as I made my way through the city. Even my

97-year old grandfather, a lifelong athlete, adamantly refuses to use a cane. "No way," he would say. How was I supposed to feel okay about it??

My cane was covered with multi-colored butterflies, mostly because I thought it was humorous. I didn't want the plain, tired looking black medical cane. I went with something that was more lighthearted. I have even had compliments on my *cane*. All these years trying to get my make up on correctly, hair done just right, clothes looking nice, and I am getting compliments on my cane?? I did finally start to realize that it wasn't the hideous, awful piece of "medical equipment" I saw it as. It wasn't something to feel humiliated and embarrassed about. It was a tool that I could use to navigate the world. It was the only reason I could actually leave the house on certain days!

I vividly recall passing by a bathroom mirror on one of the first days I used my cane in public. I felt so ancient physically. I passed by elderly patients in the hospital, we exchanged knowing smiles as we scooted past each other like snails. I made my way into the restroom, and looked at my reflection in the mirror. I recall being absolutely shocked that I looked so young. I felt at least 90 as I walked, and this reflection did not match up. I found myself spending little time looking at my face lately, being so consumed with my physical issues. I was no longer focused on trying to achieve the perfect make-up and hair I had always sought as a younger woman. Looking in that bathroom mirror, I realized that *I was still me.* I was still there, even though my body felt atrocious at times. It was a mixture of relief and disbelief, and I realized that the way I felt physically did not jive with my outward appearance. I was still young, regardless of the cane!

The fact is, assistive devices (as well as your underlying disease) do not define you as an individual. They don't tell the world who you really are, they only speak to your physical state at that moment. The more important point is that these devices can enable you to get around the world like a "normal" person, rather than remaining housebound 24 hours per day. Getting out and enjoying life is more preferable than staying home and feeling embarrassed. After all, who cares what people think? This is your life, not theirs. You may find, as I have, that using something as simple as a disabled parking placard can be met with disapproving stares. Others may not fully understand why a seemingly young, "normal" person would need to take up a parking spot meant for the disabled. I have a new mantra that passes through my mind if I feel eyes staring at me in public: "Judge away..."

No one knows anything about your struggle, your challenges, and your battle. These things are yours, this life is yours, and no one has any right to judge. Making that leap from "invisible" to publicly visible disease is a tough one, and you can anticipate very mixed feelings about it. I would recommend talking with other patients who have gone through this exact experience, and getting some suggestions. Assistive devices can be miraculous for patients who are very limited otherwise. The blue parking spaces are there for you. Try not to let your vanity keep you from enjoying your life!

The truth is, you are no longer that healthy, illness-free individual that you were before your diagnosis. You will never be that person again, but that does not mean that life is over. The process of letting go of our former selves is very difficult for many patients, but letting go is a requirement for moving forward. We cannot hang onto the past if we are to move into the future. Your past is no longer reality, and all you have is the present moment.

Embrace the present, let go of the past, and look forward to an exciting new future.

Acceptance is part of grieving, a necessary part of any loss, and it generally comes after a great deal of distress. Achieving true acceptance is a difficult process, one that is marked by a great deal of anger, sadness, denial, and pain. I had to accept my reality, because I found that if I did not, my goals were impossible to reach.

Little limitations, such as a cane, and eventually an AFO leg brace for my weakened left leg helped me to get across campus. A disabled placard allowed me to park close enough to make it to my classes on time, without the tremendous struggle. Elevators helped me by saving me the trouble of climbing flights of stairs. These tiny changes allowed me to continue on my path, regardless of my illness. They key is to start *accepting* the illness, so you can start *overcoming it.* The inner thoughts that come with this phase should be things like "It is going to be okay. I can do this. I am at peace with my reality."

Journal 5: Acceptance:

Have you reached this stage yet? Do you find yourself believing that you have a promising future, regardless of MS? Are you at peace with your diagnosis?

6

Graduation

*"However difficult life may seem, there is always
something you can do and succeed at."*
-Stephen Hawking

The day I thought would never come was here. It was a
mad rush, with all of the graduates clamoring to dress in
the deep black gowns and caps. The satiny glimmer of
these robes we had earned through years of sweat, tears,
stress, anxiety, and triumph. These orange Masters scarves,
indicative of the nursing school color, draped around our
shoulders in pride. Flashes went off throughout the room,
each graduate documenting the day with photographs that
would stand proudly in frames throughout all our homes
for generations. We looked at each other with half belief.
Were we really all here? Was this day real? It was an
utterly astounding moment to realize that nothing, not
even this disgusting, dreadful monster of a disease had
stopped me.

Many moments of the preceding 3 years flashed through my mind as I drove to the school. That phone call on the freeway where I learned my diagnosis, the sympathetic eyes of my coworkers, the hospital rooms. The infusion centers, the medications, and the relapses. The MRI images of my brain and spinal cord covered in bright white lesions, and the terror of that moment. Each event passed through my memory like a life review, all culminating in this joyous occasion.

I feared for so many years that I would be unable to walk myself down the grassy aisle. I feared that my mind would fail me, fatigue would overtake me, and my memory would not cooperate with this enormous load of learning. My fears were a major obstacle, and I doubted myself on an almost daily basis. The contemptuous voices within whispered in my ear as I attempted to walk confidently into a patient's room to play the role of provider. *"Why are you doing this? Who are you kidding? You have no business trying to do this. You are ILL."* I am not sure why they plagued me so much at this point. I suppose it was the stark realization that I had become a chronically ill patient. I had cared for so many neurological patients in my career, and most of them were incredibly debilitated. I pictured them, and I pictured my own grandmother. These were the examples of MS that I had seen previously, and those images were inescapable. It was almost as if the degree of success I experienced led to an equivalent level of negative self- talk. It took me several years to overcome this, and eventually those voices quieted. I began to meet other MS patients who were continuing with life in a variety of ways, despite MS.

I focused on those who were athletes, professionals, writers, artists, and poets. I found stories wherever I could, inspirational stories of life with MS. These became my primary focus during this difficult time, when I was walking a tiny tightrope that hung over defeat and discouragement below. At any moment, I felt that I could plummet. I knew that if I gave in to these voices, that my defeat was inevitable. I could not allow myself to be my own worst enemy. I always found it interesting that I heard no one ever discourage me, but in my own mind I had to fight discouraging myself! The most inspiring thing for many MS patients is to see a living example of success despite the illness. We can read all of the scientific texts about the causes, treatments, and diagnosis of MS, we can listen to our neurologists ramble about our EDSS scores, our physical exam, and our MRI results. These things in the end are meaningless, however. What really makes an impact is to see the individual story of another human being who has thrived with this disease. I read as many inspirational MS stories as I could get my hands on during those few years. I gobbled them up like candy, and I could not get enough. Those stories got me through some extremely difficult moments.

An important lesson I learned was that we are capable of self-defeat. It would be so much easier to quit, right? On those difficult, painful, fatigue ridden days? It is so tempting to give in and take the easy road, and many people succumb to this path. It doesn't require MS, either; many individuals find any excuse to give up. You must find that voice that *encourages* rather than *discourages.* Find that voice that will carry you through those days. Nothing worth doing is ever easy, so make the choice to be the hero of your own story. You have the ability, now all you need is to cultivate the psychological resolve.

On this day, in May of 2012, there was light. Spring, warmth, and brightly colored flowers surrounded me like a renewal, out of the cold winter and into the sun. The way the fresh grass smelled, the slow march into the ceremony, the smiles. Like a wedding or the birth of a new baby, this was a day that I would always remember, though there was also a sense of disappointment along with the accomplishment. There was a pre-graduation let down, as I knew that with the completion of this goal, I would need another. I would need a new focus to distract me from the reality that was MS. Yes, this was a successful endeavor, but what would be next? I felt my mind start to wander on to the next potential goal, but I was determined not to focus on anything but that moment. This was a day to spend celebrating, laughing, and feeling a sense of pure joy and relief. Why trouble myself with the future today? This was a day just to be present.

I felt my diagnosis and its chains drop away behind me. I could sense the snarling monsters created by my fear and anxiety slink away into the shadows, afraid of the cascading sunlight and applause that fell all around us. In that moment, my hand reached out to shake the University President's. My family members smiled from rows away, and time stood still. The diploma was passed, and my grip did not fail me. For in that moment, I was free.

In that moment, I was *me.*

As I walked with my family through that beautiful campus, I knew it would be the last time I would visit here as a student. I looked over my shoulder behind me as I drove away, and I realized that this was a beautiful chapter of my life that was coming to a close. But, as they say, when one door closes another opens, only this time, *I* closed the door, not my disease.

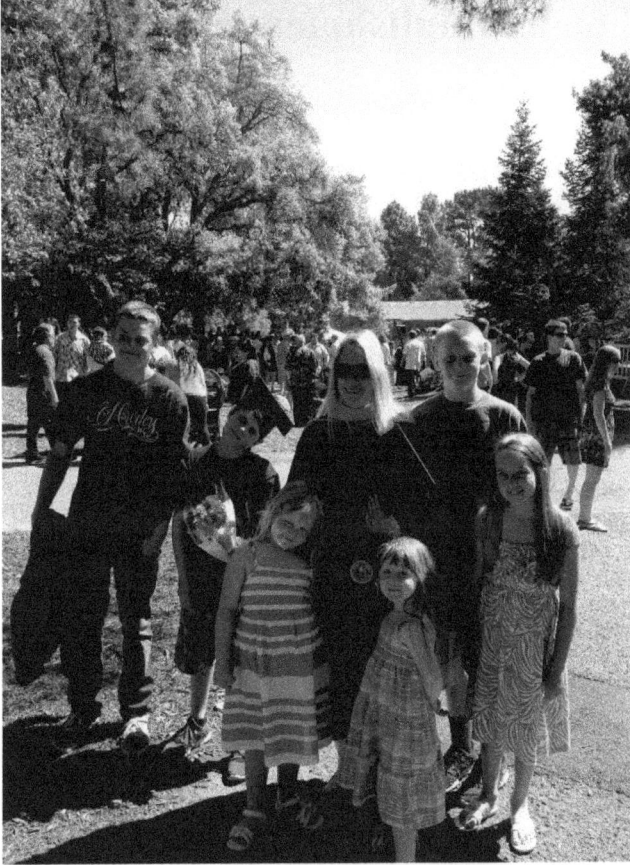

Masters graduation, 2012

Journal 6: Accomplishments:

What have you accomplished since your diagnosis? Have you learned to somehow ignore those demotivating voices in your head? How have you learned to overcome your adversities, and what would you tell someone who is newly diagnosed?

PART TWO: IDENTITY CRISIS

7

Patient and Healer

"The art of medicine consists in amusing the patient while nature cures the disease"
-Voltaire

After my graduation from Sonoma State University in 2012, I immediately went to work as Family Nurse Practitioner in a local family practice and sports medicine office. With that success, I felt so encouraged. I now knew I could succeed despite this diagnosis, it did not change who I was, and I could overcome. No one in the office knew of my diagnosis initially, and I loved that. It was almost like playing a role: The strong, capable primary care provider. I enjoyed the fact that I could successfully perform my duties despite MS, and my patients seemed to really like me! My days were long and very difficult at times. As anyone with MS knows, there are definite "good" days and distinct "bad" days. These are unpredictable changes, and I had to get up each morning and put my patient's needs before my own.

I absolutely loved my new work. I was independent finally, which is what I hoped to achieve by becoming a provider. I had hundreds of patients in my list of regulars. I performed exams, physicals, ordered diagnostic tests and prescribed medications. I was the dependable healthcare professional, and I was always ready to help when my patients needed me most. I diagnosed and treated minor and major illnesses, referred to specialists, and provided a shoulder to cry on for many patients over the course of years. Unlike my previous position as an ER RN, I was now the primary health provider for my patients. I was alone in that room, with no one to help me. This was frightening at first, but I grew more accustomed to the role as time went on. My confidence grew, and I knew I could perform my duties skillfully and successfully.

I worked for a wonderful, small practice with just one other physician. He was a great mentor, and was always happy to lend an opinion when needed. Those moments when a patient stumped me, confused me, or presented with a problem I had never seen before, my physician co-worker would happily step in the room. The staff members in the office were supportive and kind, and I could not believe I had been so blessed to find them. Seeing my name on a prescription pad, a business card, and online advertisements for the office was exhilarating and unforgettable. I felt I had achieved the success that I had strived so long for. This was what I had dreamed of for so many years.

Being a healthcare provider is a selfless, often thankless job. Frequently, the days of seeing family practice patients can be monotonous. You get into a rhythm, and the management of diabetes, high blood pressure, and high cholesterol become a daily practice.

I was supposed to be dependable, reliable and confident, yet MS doesn't always cooperate with that image does it? This dichotomy was a struggle for me, and continues to be. What different roles, patient and provider. Being ill was not part of my plan, but as human beings we are incredibly good at adapting to our circumstances. I found myself developing a split personality, and I am sure everyone with MS can relate to this.

I started to experience the irony of my situation. I was supposed to be the healer, yet I was ill. I was supposed to be the provider, but I was the patient at the same time.

In primary care, many patients have very minor issues to discuss, such as sore throats, common colds, and wart removal. Many patients asked for work excuses for issues I felt were very minor. At times I felt like saying: "I am sicker than YOU are," but I resisted the urge. Some patients were far worse off, suffering from diabetes, heart disease, and pulmonary issues. I felt so connected to those with chronic ailments. I knew what it was like to carry the burden of an incurable disease, and I struggled with the decision to share my own experience with my patients, it just felt unprofessional. Would they still have faith in me as a provider if they knew I had MS? Would they leave my practice to see another provider who wasn't sick? Would their trust in me fade a bit if they knew?

My situation was unique, and it was a daily struggle. I asked myself: Would I want a provider who truly understood my experience? Of course I would. We don't often consider our providers when we go in for an appointment. We are so focused on our own issues, the questions we want answered, and the treatments we need. It isn't natural to consider the human being that is treating us. Who are they? Are they having a good day, or a bad one? Are they ill themselves? These are questions that never crossed my mind before I stood in their shoes. Did anyone even consider who I was?

Being a primary care provider, I began to really know every detail of my patient's lives, and it is a balance between sharing and listening. I began to develop a sense of my patient's needs and personalities, and I knew which patients would benefit from hearing my story. I would share my story, and some of my chronically ill patients felt so relieved to know that I truly understood. I was anxious to share too much, but I found that the patients who needed to feel that someone truly cared and really *got it* were grateful.

It is an isolating experience at times, being chronically ill, and some of my patients had no friends and family to speak to. I was the sole source of emotional and physical support for these patients, and some patients would make appointments simply to talk. I find that some providers are cold and distant, only seeing patients as a disease process. What about the mind? We are so much more than a body. Providers should always see the patient as a mind-body unit, addressing the full scope of chronic illness. Psychological and emotional symptoms are common, and no one should leave an appointment feeling dismissed.

As I have mentioned, I am a classically trained, western medical health professional. I am not a physician, however, I am a nurse practitioner. We are trained a bit differently than physicians, and in a way that I feel is more holistic. We are trained from day one to see the humanistic side of medicine, to view the patient as a whole being, rather than the sum of the parts. The body cannot be healed without addressing the spiritual, emotional aspects of the human being. After being diagnosed with a chronic illness, I appreciated this manner of teaching more than ever before.

There is an intricate, indivisible connection between the body and the mind, and treating only one while ignoring the other will never prove effective. There is, what we call in medicine, an "emotional overlay," to almost every physical issue. Whether this means that the condition is purely psychological, or whether the mind is reacting to a physical issue (anxiety, panic attacks, depression,) the mind must always be taken into consideration when treating every patient.

The human body is an amazing machine, and with great consistency, it works flawlessly. Many people live their lives to the ripe old age of 80 something, without any major medical problems. Most medical issues will simply resolve on their own regardless of treatment. Sinusitis, ear infections, minor lacerations, viral illnesses such as colds/flu, and seasonal allergies are self-limiting, and the body is excellent at healing. These issues *almost always* resolve with what we refer to as "tincture of time." People do not like to accept that answer, however. Many want an immediate, quick and easy fix.

Our society is very quick to assume that modern medicine has all the answers, a secret book of treatments, available only to those who have attended medical school. This magic book contains all of the recipes for treating illness, and is kept hidden, under lock and key. The providers of the world are assumed to have the ability to fix anything, treat anything, and if they do not offer a fix, they are assumed to be withholding treatment intentionally.

I can tell you, this is not the case. One of the most shocking things I learned while transitioning from a registered nurse to a nurse practitioner was the absolute limitation in options we have as providers. We only have a few things to offer, a few laboratory tests, an x-ray or two, a few medications that may or may not be effective. Most medications also go along with an enormous list of potential side effects that have to be taken into consideration. Many prescription medications are not necessary, and can lead to a variety of new problems. The risk versus the benefit of any treatment needs to be considered. Treating physical illness is not only a science, but also an art. Sometimes, treatment is experimental, or anecdotal. Sometimes, providers simply run out of ideas. Every possible treatment option has been exhausted, and there is simply nothing further to offer. I find that patients are shocked when this is the answer. "What do you mean, there is nothing left to do?" Sometimes, the answer is just that, and the patient is left with trying to cope with their "new normal." Whether that means pain, numbness, weakness, or any other symptom.

We are making progress in many areas of medicine, but we are still far from being able to treat many conditions effectively enough. MS is a wonderful example of this. MS, and many other autoimmune diseases such as type 1 diabetes and lupus remain major medical mysteries.

We have come a long way, but we haven't gone far enough. We have our handful of treatment options for RRMS, but the benefits are not incredibly impressive from a statistical standpoint. Reduction of relapses at about 30-50% is the most we can hope for, but this is a vast improvement over the "zero options" that my grandmother had. Treatments for progressive MS are still badly lacking, and my hope is that this will be the focus of new research.

When you visit your provider, keep in mind that they may not have an answer for every question you have. Your provider is doing their best, I am sure; but the answer "I do not know," is an acceptable one sometimes. I always trust providers who admit that they do not have an answer, because this is honesty. If your provider says, "Well, if you really want to take something you can try this..." this is code for- "you really do not need this." Sometimes, in medicine, less is best. The minimalist approach to treatment is wise, and so many patients have been "overtreated" in recent years. Too many medications, wasteful, unnecessary diagnostic testing, and the resulting side effects and anxiety are major issues in medicine currently. Patients and providers need to take a moment and ask themselves, "Is this really a necessary test or treatment?"

Trust your body to be able to handle most minor issues. Your body is an intricate, well-constructed, dynamic machine that is much wiser than we are as health providers. Now and then, the body might need an extra hand at combating an infection, but not always. Listen to your body! Prevention is the key! Get your immunizations, get some exercise, eat healthy foods, and obviously avoid smoking and alcohol. MS aside, we all need the same basic advice on remaining healthy and living the best life possible.

Questions to Ask Your Provider at Appointments:

1. **Do you feel that my disease is well controlled with my current medication?**
2. **If not, are there other medications available that you would recommend?**
3. **Do you recommend any other treatments for my current symptoms (alternative or traditional?)**
4. **How often do you recommend appointments and MRI?**

5. Is there any new research that has become available since my last appointment?

Disease-Modifying therapies are one of the main topics of discussion between an MS patient and their providers. These are difficult choices to make, and the opinions may vary between providers. These drugs are powerful, may have significant side effects, and can be incredibly costly. I received my shipment of Tecfidera today from FedEx, and with it, I received my usual receipt and medication instructions. I receive one month of medication at a time, via FedEx. Today, I stopped to read the receipt.

"Your drug benefit saved you: $5290.55."

Keep in mind, this was for one month of Tecfidera. This really got me thinking about the state of our health care system, our "for-profit" drug companies, and the seemingly unaffordable, astronomical cost of our multiple sclerosis drugs. We can always talk at length about politics, health care affordability and accessibility, and the laws governing those things. However, in the forefront of my mind are those MS patients who have no ability to afford these medications. Most Americans do not earn $5290 per month, let alone have the ability to pay for these drugs.

According to the Social Security Administration, the average income in the US in 2012 was $44,321 (SSA.gov.)

Multiple Sclerosis is a unique disease, as far as medications go. The disease is currently incurable, and does not tend to shorten the lifespan very much. This leads to the demand for lifelong medication treatment, and a large profit for drug companies. The ethics of this situation are debatable. I am one of the lucky ones, because I am fortunate enough to be insured. I pay 5$ per month instead of $5000. I want so much to help those who aren't as lucky.

I was pleased to discover that all approved disease-modifying medications have prescription assistance programs. I want to share some important drug assistance resources with my fellow MS patients, and hope these will be helpful to anyone who needs these programs. As we know, disease-modifying drugs are extremely important in our arsenal of treatments for this disease:

Aubagio
Program name: MS One 2 One
Phone: (855) 676-6326
Website: www.aubagio.com

Avonex
Program name: MS ActiveSource
Phone: (800) 456-2255
Website: www.avonex.com

Betaseron
Program name: BetaPlus
Phone: (800) 788-1467
Website: www.betaseron.com

Copaxone
Program name: Shared Solutions
Phone: (800) 887-8100
Website: www.copaxone.com

Extavia
Patient Services Program
Phone: (866) 398-2842
Website: www.extavia.com

Gilenya
Patient Services Program
Phone: (800) 445-3692
Website: www.gilenya.com

Plegridy
Program name: MS ActiveSource
Phone: (800) 456-2255
Website: plegridy.com

Rebif
Program name: MS Lifelines
Phone: (877) 447-3243
Website: www.mslifelines.com

Tecfidera
Program name: MS ActiveSource
Phone: (800) 456-2255
Website: www.tecfidera.com

Tysabri
Program name: MS ActiveSource
Phone: (800) 456-2255
Website: www.tysabri.com

If your physician has prescribed one of these medications, and you are unable to afford the cost, do not give up. Please try to reach out to one of these assistance programs, and remember that there are resources available for those in need. Never give up, and find a provider who truly understands. Find a provider who truly believes that the idea is to care for the physical body, while also supporting human being within.

Journal 7: Your Healthcare Provider:

Have you found a provider you feel fully comfortable with? Can you openly express your feelings and needs? If not, what would your ideal provider be like?

8

Hypervigilance: Predicting the Unpredictable

"We must let go of the life we have planned, so as to accept the one that is waiting for us."
-Joseph Campbell

Hypervigilance.

"Abnormally increased responsiveness to stimuli, and scanning of the environment for threats."

The longer I live with this label of MS, the more convinced I become that the most difficult and life-altering consequence of this disease is the constant awareness of its existence. I have relapsing-remitting MS, and the very essence of my disease involves periods of relapse, with severe symptoms that affect my entire world, followed inexplicably by periods of near remission. It is something you slowly learn to live with, uncertainty, but it never becomes normal. It is almost like being robbed of your innocence, your ability to feel at ease is taken forever. Even in periods of relative remission, a dark cloud of uncertainty followed me.

A state of alertness is designed to protect us from threats and danger, and it serves a much-needed purpose in those situations. When we are in an acutely dangerous environment, we must have the ability to respond. Imagine being in a life-threatening situation: A wild animal is chasing us, a maniac is trying to kill us, etc. What happens? Our bodies prepare for a fight for life, the "fight or flight" response. Our heart rates increase, our respiratory rate increases, our blood pressure rises, and our pupils dilate to allow us to respond to the impending destructive force headed our way.

What happens when we are in this state of alertness and vigilance for an extended period of time? In the case of multiple sclerosis, we are in this state for the rest of our lives. We never have a day without this monkey on our backs. Never again (without an absolute cure) will we feel utterly at ease.

Extended periods of hypervigilance will eventually lead to secondary problems. The main issues become anxiety, insomnia, fatigue, and social withdrawal/seclusion. Many MS patients begin to withdraw from normal social circles, becoming overly focused on the disease in exchange for formally enjoyable activities. This experience can be even more devastating than the physical symptoms.

Symptoms of Anxiety

- **Feeling nervous or excessively worrying**
- **Feeling hopeless or out of control**
- **Having a sense of impending danger, panic or doom**
- **Increased heart rate**
- **Rapid breathing (hyperventilation)**
- **Increased Sweating**
- **Shaking or Trembling**
- **Fatigue or inability to sleep**
- **Trouble concentrating and hypervigilance (constant scanning of environment for threats)**

I found that I would wake up in that early morning haze, just barely conscious from my sleep, feeling peaceful from my last dream, and immediately upon opening my eyes it was as if a voice would scream into my ear, "YOU HAVE MS!!!!!" I would feel my heart start to race, I would sit upright, and the crushing blow of diagnosis would sink in yet again. This experience repeated itself daily for the first couple of years post diagnosis. It was very hard for me to communicate this experience to anyone I knew. I had no close friends with MS, and I did not believe my family would understand. Soon, I became obsessed with scanning my sensory experiences, looking for a new symptom. Each day, there was something new. A new buzzing sensation, a new numb area, a new area of skin that felt "sunburned" and painful, and several times, new onset of blurry and dim vision. I have lost much of my vision in the last 5 years. I went from having 20/20 vision 5 years ago, to 20/100 today due to repeated bouts with optic neuritis.

When you live with a daily fear of new deficits, you change. It is difficult to fall asleep at night thinking, "What new symptom will I wake up with tomorrow?" How do you live your life? How do you plan your work, your children's activities, or your driving? The key is to plan for the worst, and hope for the best. After the diagnosis of MS, we live with a lifetime of unpredictability. It is a way of life, and it is something we all must adjust to. Many of us like to carry on like brave soldiers, but in the end it is sometimes better to plan for the worst and be happy if it isn't that bad after all.

In my work as a nurse practitioner, I started to experience an extension of my hypervigilance with my patients. I would see a patient in that magic 20-40 year age bracket, complaining of neurologic symptoms such as numbness, fatigue, balance issues, or visual deficits, and I would feel that familiar sense of dread. I would immediately think: "Oh God what if this is MS?" When patients complained of inexplicable, full-body pain, I immediately thought of Fibromyalgia. When patients complained of joint pain, Rheumatoid Arthritis popped into my mind instantly. I found myself leaping to conclusions in my practice, mostly because of my own experience. I would jump to conclusions too quickly, and I could sense that I was becoming biased and non-objective in these cases. I often hear other chronically ill patients describe the years of struggle to obtain a diagnosis, and I shudder.

The early symptoms of many chronic diseases can mimic other conditions, and it can be extremely difficult for providers to determine the cause. Obviously, I could not simply order an MRI for every patient who complained of blurry vision, bladder issues, or balance problems. I had to rule out the more common reasons for these problems first. When most providers see a relatively young, healthy patient complain of these symptoms, 99% of the time the patient will not have a serious condition. It is important for patients to remain insistent, return for visits, document and inform the provider of every one of them. Often, seeing a cluster of symptoms persisting over time is more of a clue.

I was a firm believer in getting a diagnosis as quickly as possible for my patients so that treatment could be initiated rapidly. This was also difficult as a provider, because I understood that once that diagnosis was made, my patient would also go through this life altering change. How could I lead a patient through the process of diagnosis, knowing what was waiting at the end? I spent a great deal of time seeking advice from other NPs and physicians, trying to overcome this. I learned to manage it, but the worry was always present.

Here is the good news: You can learn to manage this issue. If you find yourself staying home rather than enjoying your normal activities, losing sleep worrying about your illness, feeling tremendous anxiety, or any other life-altering symptom, get help. Sometimes it is as simple as finding the right support group. Sometimes individual or group counseling is helpful. The point is, don't just suffer alone needlessly. And most importantly: Don't feel like you are "crazy." You aren't!

With many chronic illnesses, you have periods of relative normalcy. Sometimes you even start to believe that you are 100% healthy again during a long period of remission. But then, you are attacked again when you least expect it. Human beings need an element of predictability in life, and without it, we go a little crazy. The inability to predict the immediate future leads to a myriad of issues, and we tend to become hopeless and generally apathetic when we feel there is no way to control our lives. This apathy is a dangerous thing, and can lead to many other issues down the road.

Studies have been done on primates and *learned helplessness*: "Learned helplessness, in psychology, a mental state in which an organism forced to bear aversive stimuli, or stimuli that are painful or otherwise unpleasant, becomes unable or unwilling to avoid subsequent encounters with those stimuli, even if they are "escapable," presumably because it has learned that it cannot control the situation" (Encyclopedia Britannica, 2014.) In essence, living creatures stop trying to avoid unpleasant stimuli all together if they feel that they have no control. The will to fight and avoid pain is gone, and they become entirely helpless.

It's not as if we can control our flares. The idea is: If we learn that we cannot control our lives, we develop an attitude of helplessness. We give up even trying to live or control any aspect of our lives. This is the source of the anxiety and depression that so often accompany the disease. Fighting that constant, daily knowledge of our utter lack of control over our own bodies is a difficult predicament. In my own life, the challenge was to practice a daily mantra of, "It could always be worse." We all have different approaches when it comes to coping with difficult life situations. In the face of adversity, my Grandfather's response was an unyielding defiance, exemplified by his favorite poem, *Invictus.*

This poem meant so much to him, and it sat in his home, on display, serving as a daily reminder to him during the most difficult times. At the end of his life, it was fittingly read during his memorial service.

Invictus

BY WILLIAM ERNEST HENLEY

Out of the night that covers me,

Black as the pit from pole to pole,

I thank whatever gods may be

For my unconquerable soul.

In the fell clutch of circumstance

I have not winced nor cried aloud.

Under the bludgeonings of chance

My head is bloody, but unbowed.

Beyond this place of wrath and tears

Looms but the Horror of the shade,

And yet the menace of the years

Finds and shall find me unafraid.

It matters not how strait the gate,

How charged with punishments the scroll,

I am the master of my fate,

I am the captain of my soul.

This is a depiction of one form of coping during challenging times, and it inspires me to read it today, many years after his death. The attitude of many of my family members is that no matter how difficult life might become, we have ultimate control over our fear, anxiety, and worry. We cannot necessarily control what fate has in store for us, but we definitely do not need to spend every single day terrified of the possibilities, do we?

In the face of struggle, tragedy, and challenge, we always have the option to be strong in spite of it. This manner of thinking allows us to feel that we have some element of control over our circumstances, especially when we feel that life has started to spin out of control. We can always choose how we *react* to life's challenges. Our reaction is the only thing we can ultimately control, every single time.

Anxiety is a distressing affliction, one that I have suffered from during these past 5 years. If anything in life challenges my ability to cope with worry, MS does. As patients, we live with utter and complete uncertainty from the moment of diagnosis. These diseases have such a vast array of possible courses, so how can we possibly know what *our own* course will be? The range runs the gamut from almost zero symptoms, to total disability.

The answer is, we don't know. We look to our medical professionals to try to predict our outcomes, but they cannot at this point. Medical science has grown highly skilled at diagnosing these conditions, but less skilled at letting us know what to expect. For example, all forms of MS generally appear the same way at diagnosis, with lesions on MRI and physical symptoms, often with abnormalities of the cerebrospinal fluid. There is no known way to predict the course this illness will take after that point.

This leaves us, as patients, with no choice but to take life day by day. For the first couple of years after diagnosis, I was at my wit's end with anxiety. I was a natural "control freak," so this disease tested my ability to cope with the unknown. Over the course of time, we start to become more comfortable with our version of the disease, and more able to predict our own illness. This is our ultimate opportunity to listen to those numerous inspirational quotes that advise us to "live in the moment." Before MS, I used to overlook these things and think, "Yeah yeah, live in the moment. I get it." Now, I began to stop and really ponder what that meant.

Stop focusing on what could go wrong, and start trying to focus on what could go right. The fact of the matter is, no human being on the planet can predict what even the next hour will bring. Having a chronic illness makes our life no more uncertain than anyone else's. We have simply had the curtain pulled back, and we can see the truth behind it. We have the opportunity to appreciate the uncertainty of life more than those who are healthy. We are acutely, sometimes painfully aware of the limitations of life, and I believe that this is actually a blessing in disguise. This awareness allows us the chance to not just read the quotes, but to live them; and to actually, truthfully, honestly *be in the moment*.

The line of the poem "under the bludgeonings of chance," refers to the completely unpredictable nature of our lives. This unpredictability is the cause of anxiety for so many people, especially those carrying the burden of MS. Our lives are indeed unpredictable, there is no arguing that point, but in the end, we are all the masters of our fate. Regardless of your disease course, don't ever feel like you can't steer your own life in the direction you want it to go.

I tried to challenge myself to look outward when I was overly focused inward on my own troubles. Looking outward, even reading the newspaper or watching network news for five minutes was often enough to snap me out of my dark place. The suffering in this world is extreme, and was my suffering any worse than anyone's? Not really. War, starvation, disease, poverty, oppression. The list goes on and on. If I practiced *gratitude* I could always pull myself up and out of the pity party. It was difficult to spend much time feeling sorry for myself as a mother of six. I needed to get up, be present, and care for others on a daily basis. Having someone to care for is very helpful for me. Whether it is a pet, child, or friend, if someone is depending on you, it forces you to look outward.

Suggestions for managing the unpredictable nature of MS

1. Get to know your body.

Learn to be sensitive to the subtle, early signs of a relapse and *slow down.*

2. Avoid stress as much as possible.

Go get a massage, do yoga, have acupuncture, meditate, breathe, or practice guided relaxation.

3. Educate yourself.

Learn as much as you can about your individual disease, and you will feel more in control.

4. Find an excellent provider you can call/email at the drop of a hat.

Find someone you feel is responsive and ready to help you when the next relapse strikes. If you have confidence in your provider, you will feel more in control.

5. Have a support system.

Have a network of friends, family, caregivers, and resources. Make connections. Online, by phone, or in person. Attend a support group, or an online chat. Keep yourself connected so that you will never feel alone.

Remember, you are strong and capable. Repeat that mantra:

IT COULD ALWAYS BE WORSE!

Sometimes, I just want to hear reality, don't you? I want to hear that I am not insane, that this is real, and others are going through similar experiences. Connecting through mutual struggle is something I find incredibly necessary in the case of any chronic condition. I am hopeful that sharing my own experience will help someone out there having a particularly difficult day.

Journal 8: Hypervigilance? Anxiety?

Have you had symptoms such as worrying, scanning for new symptoms excessively, or full-blown anxiety and panic attacks? How do you cope? Have you found any techniques that work for these symptoms?

9

A Stolen Memory: Parents With MS

"Every child begins the world again."
-Henry David Thoreau

How will my children remember me?

Isn't that a question every parent asks? We want to set the best example for our kids, leaving a legacy behind when we are gone. Often, this is one of the main reasons people choose to become parents in the first place. One of the first fears in the minds of parents who are diagnosed with a chronic illness is: "How will this disease affect my ability to parent?" Followed soon by, "Will my young children remember me when I was healthy?" Illnesses often strike in the prime of adulthood, when most people are finally successful in a career, finally married, or starting new families. This is the cruelest aspect of these illnesses, the theft of young optimism.

We want our children to recall these years of health, vitality, energy and strength. We want them to remember vacations, playing ball, swimming, and dancing with us. We want them to remember us as young, beautiful adults who never failed them. Illness interferes with that image, and creates an image of inability, dependence, and weakness. Struggle and sadness replace happiness and health, failure and decline replace the image of success and achievement.

I was diagnosed with MS after the birth of my fifth and final child, and I often spend time thinking, "Would I have had all these children if I had known?" Unlikely. I would have been better prepared to *slow down* my life as much as possible and brace for the future. I would have had more time to rest in the quiet and recover from my relapses. I would have had more time to spend taking care of myself instead of my large family. My days generally go like this (does this sound anything like YOUR day??):

6:45 am: The alarm sounds rhythmically, like an unseen hand smacking me across the face. Pulling me from the peaceful slumber and dream world I had been roaming, without a care. In the dream, I was whole, I was energetic, young and beautiful. In the dream I had no numbness, weakness, or dim vision. I also had no fear.

"MOM! She's HITTING ME!!!" A voice from the other room bellows, the first of a million little arguments I will have to referee today. My left arm feels weak. I don't remember that yesterday. My right leg is tingling, and that hasn't happened in some time. What does this mean? Is this a new relapse?

7:00am: The dog is whining again. What does he want now? "STOP WEARING MY CLOTHES!!" The voice has the tone of two iron pots banging together in my ear. Ah yes, another argument. My left arm is noticeably weaker than it was yesterday, and I just know another relapse has started. It has only been 2 months since I had steroids last, and it is probably too soon to do them again. The steroids, that make me feel insane, make my face bloat, and my hair fall out. Those lovely things. "MOM I am HUNGRY!!"

8:00am: Driving the kids to school, vision is blurry. Eyes are dim, and my focus is difficult to keep. My left hand trembles noticeably as I grip the wheel. Should I call someone to help drive? Is this even safe? My God. How is this my life? "STOP LOOKING AT ME LIKE THAT! YOU'RE **MEAN**," echoes from the tiny mouth to her sister in the back seat.

9:00 am: Home from the drop offs (5 kids, 4 different schools.) I stop to glance in the mirror briefly. I look like I have climbed out of some deep, dank tomb somewhere. What happened to me? My hair is in clumps. I have no time for this! This hand. It's definitely weak. Off to call the neurologist. What will this mean? Is my medicine no longer working? This is the fifth medication I have tried. How many more will I need to try? Will any of them ever work?

10:00 am: I have once again forgotten to take my six morning pills. Now I am taking them late. Why don't I ever learn? I need to start writing things down. My memory is horrendous. The phone rings. Is that the neurologist calling back? I am losing more and more grip with this left hand, and my eye is DEFINITELY worse. "Hello, this is your daughter's school. She's in the office with a 101 degree temperature and she just vomited. You need to come get her." Again, how is this my life??

12:00 pm: The child is vomiting. Repeatedly. Oh, and having diarrhea. Lucky me. I am sure I will be next. The phone rings, it's the neurologist. "Do you want steroids, then?" He says. "That's what I can offer you." Oh, Joy. Another 3 days in and out of the infusion center.

2:00pm: My mother comes to help me with the vomiting child, and I am driving myself to the hospital for the first of three days of steroid infusions. The other children are done with school in one hour, so I hope its fast.

My left hand is incredibly weak, and my vision has decreased tremendously since this morning.

3:00 pm: They found a vein on the first stick, and I sat, listening to the click-clicking of the IV pump as the infusion made its way into my arm. I made small talk with the nurses, who were almost all my former coworkers. I recall when I was one of them. I used to be the one starting the IVs. It is hitting me now: I am ILL.

4:00pm: Home, and all kids picked up. IV left in place for tomorrow's infusion. "MOM!!!! I'M HUNGRY!!!!!" scream the kids. What the hell am I going to serve these kids for dinner? My husband is working until midnight as an ER physician, so I am on my own until then. I guess it's delivery pizza again!! They must think I am insane at the pizza place.

6:00 pm: Is it me, or has the volume of homework increased ten-fold since I was in school? Why does every child have an essay due tomorrow? "MOM!! SHE HIT ME AGAIN!!" Boy the steroids are really hitting me now. I am going to LOSE IT!

8:00 pm: Kids bathed. Homework done? I am flying like I have had 10,000 cups of coffee, and the IV left in my arm was a bad idea. The youngest nearly yanked it out twice. 2 are in bed, 4 are still awake. Most of the homework is done. 2 are fighting over the TV, and 2 massive teenage boys are consuming every single thing I have in the kitchen in a furious late night eating rampage. Boy, my vision is BAD.

10:00 pm: There is no way I am going to sleep tonight. I will need to take something. This is too much. Everyone has finally quieted down, and my mind is running a marathon. Every single philosophical thought you can imagine is streaming through my steroid soaked brain, pondering the mysteries of the universe. "WHY ME" is a particularly interesting subject at this point. Well, off to sleep in a haze. I Have to be up at 6:45 am to do it all over again........

Sound familiar? I am sure most parents can relate to this. We never get a moment, and we never get a break. Sick days are not an option for parents, and the pay is not very good, either. We are forced to be utterly and completely selfless, from the moment these precious bundles of joy appear in our lives. Every parent is faced with this challenge, even the parents with MS. Some choose to become parents before MS ever strikes, and others choose to start or add to a family even after the diagnosis. I have great respect for patients who knowingly choose to become parents after diagnosis, because these parents are aware of exactly the challenges they will be facing with the endeavor. Those of us who stumbled upon the diagnosis long after having children do not ever have to face such a difficult decision.

Time after time, I came to the conclusion, however; that my children were the reason I got out of bed on some days. On those very difficult, dark days when every single step was a marathon, every twist of the spine was painful, and my hands wouldn't cooperate with the simplest of tasks, I would likely have just stayed in bed if it weren't for them. I recognized that I could not blame myself for the choices I made in my life. Yes, my life may have been easier without my "bunch," but easier isn't necessarily *better*. Rather than giving in and giving up on hard days, I had no choice but to get up and *try: and sometimes that's all we need.*

My grandmother had seven children during her life, and the oldest children recall her vividly as an energetic, beautiful woman with strength, endurance and a zest for life. The younger children, who were born when the decline had set in, may not have the same image in their memories. This is the true tragedy of illness, the highway robbery of our children's recollections of their parents. The responsibility of passing on memories is left to the healthy spouse, friends, and other relatives. Photographs became an essential part of life for my grandfather, and he spent many days documenting the important life events for future generations. My grandfather was also a writer, and he spent months writing a 300-page manuscript detailing the life they shared before MS. These photographs and written memories are priceless for my grandmother's children and grandchildren, those of us who never knew her when she was well. I imagine my grandmother would never want us to remember her only when she was ill. She was an amazing woman, a veteran of WWII, and world traveler. She was so much more than MS.

Those who have not experienced chronic illness greatly underestimate the social impacts. The physical symptoms (which can be absolutely devastating) are only one portion of the true impact. The stolen identities, the lost vitality, and the lost memories of parents and grandparents are incredibly painful. My own experience with MS has shown me that chronic illness is sometimes a slow torment, taking almost imperceptible pieces of me away as the days roll on. Each day brought a new loss, and with many cognitive and memory changes, I wondered if I was slowly becoming a different person altogether. Would anyone remember me as I used to be?

Photographs are amazing things. We take pictures to document our life experiences and remember particular, specific moments we would otherwise forget. Photos are a powerful way to create and establish memories, never to be forgotten. My grandfather's hundreds of photographs lived in a dark closet for many years after he passed away, and I was determined to take them out, scan them, and share them. These are virtual memories of time standing still, recollections of the way things were on one second of one minute of one day, many years ago. Priceless, lost moments we cannot retrieve.

I would advise every patient to begin "life documentation" after diagnosis. If you enjoy art, draw your memories. If you enjoy taking photographs, document every moment. If you are a writer, write your heart out until you have purged every thought and emotion onto paper. These are the memories your children, family, and friends will be able to see forever. These will live on always, no matter what life brings, for generations to come.

Just think how wonderful it would be if we had these things from our grandparents and great-grandparents; if we could hold a manuscript in our hands that was written decades ago by our loved ones? If we could hold a book of photos taken by them? If we could hold a piece of artwork done by their hand? These objects would be invaluable, priceless.

Parenting with a chronic illness is an incredibly difficult task. We must care for ourselves while simultaneously caring for our children, and it is never a simple thing. We often question how much information should be shared with our children about our illness. Should we hide the symptoms to protect them? This is probably not the best approach. Children are not as fragile as you might believe, and honesty is typically best when dealing with kids. They want to know the truth about your illness. If you do not provide a truthful description of the disease, (it is not fatal, it is not going to kill mom, but it will make her tired, weak, numb, in pain, etc.) children may conjure a terrifying fear of the illness. They may begin to believe that mom or dad is going to die, and this is not what we want them thinking. Providing an honest, truthful description of the way you feel, combined with a general, simple description of what your specific illness actually *is* might be the best approach.

Having a back-up plan in case of relapses or other urgent issues is essential for parents. You may feel that you can care for your children at all times, but chronic illness is unpredictable. There may be moments that you need a helping hand, a ride, or other household assistance. It is very important to have a list of friends, family, or other caregivers who will be there to help in case you need it. Knowing that you have this extra help available when needed will ease your anxiety, and allow you to be at peace a bit more. If you are unable to work as much as you did previously, you may find that you can truly be there for your children when they need you. Volunteering in classrooms, going along as a chaperone for field trips, or simply spending time at home with your children may all be possibilities even if your disease course has worsened. Your children want you to be present, even if you are physically weakened. Focus on the things you *can* do, rather than the things you *can't.*

Remember that honesty is always the best route with kids. You should not minimize your illness, but rather explain it in an age-appropriate manner. Let your children in on your symptoms, if you feel that would help. Hiding your illness or your frustration is never useful. You will find that your children are excellent observers, who are able to pick up on the slightest hint of distress in their parents. I believe that it is always better to share openly than to hide these things. After all, this is a part of who you are, and they love *you*. No matter how well you think you are hiding your symptoms, your disease is not going away. It is important to let your children in on this part of your life, allowing them an opportunity to process it themselves. You may have spent time processing and grieving, but your children deserve that same chance. Unless you honestly divulge your illness, this process never has a chance to occur.

It was absolutely essential to me that my children recall the happy moments: The laughter, the smiles, the joy and the love, the holidays, the vacations, the birthdays, and the major life accomplishments. These were the events that needed to be remembered and celebrated. With these written and photographic memories, we each have the opportunity to be part of the history of our families. We have the chance to be heroic in the eyes of the people who mean the most to us, for generations to come.

Important Tips For Parents With MS

1. Have a back-up plan in place for childcare and housekeeping in case of a relapse (or on particularly difficult symptom days.)

2. Be honest with your children. Let them know the truth about the illness you are battling.

3. Give your children an age-appropriate description of your illness and the symptoms.

4. If you are fatigued, try to spend time at home doing activities with the kids, such as games, small cooking projects, and art.

5. If you find yourself out of work or disabled, try volunteering in classrooms occasionally, or spending a bit more time one-on-one with your children, enjoy more "quality time."

6. Document your happy times with either photographs or written words. Let your children know how much fun you had together during childhood. Happy memories will last a lifetime.

7. Remember that even if you aren't feeling your best, your presence at family events or in the home is what is important. You do not have to be perfect, but being present makes a huge difference in your children's lives.

Journal 9: Parenting:

What has been the most difficult part of parenting since your MS diagnosis? What techniques have you found helpful? What would you tell your children if they were reading your thoughts years from now?

10

The Monster in the Mirror: Fatigue and Emotional Manifestations of MS

"We can never obtain peace in the outer world until we make peace with ourselves." -Dalai Lama

Sometimes, a monster showed itself when I was least expecting it. A snarling, growling, terrifying creature that I did not recognize, a facet of my soul that I would rather not accept as being a part of me. Yet, it was. This unrecognizable ghoul was not some character from a horror movie, not a stranger lurking outside, not a predator stalking me. This creature sat with me, right in my own home, and it fed on my anger.

I had six healthy kids, a husband who loved me, and an amazing support system. Now and then though, my resident monster made an appearance. This anger was a product of a life full of stress and responsibility, parenthood, and multiple sclerosis. Often, emotional disturbances are an early symptom of MS, and can be misdiagnosed. My grandmother had early emotional disturbances before her diagnosis in the 1950s, and MS was not diagnosed until years later. These emotional outbursts were initially diagnosed as a psychiatric condition, leading to extremely long hospital stays and inappropriate treatment. Almost every MS patient I have interviewed has complained of some type of mood disorder, ranging from mild anxiety to major depressive disorder. Mood disturbances are a rarely discussed, yet common symptom of MS.

Mood disturbances are not something many people like to openly divulge. We like to think of it as something to be afraid of, ashamed of, and hidden away. My feelings were: If I shared my own experiences with anger, frustration, anxiety, and sadness, maybe someone in my shoes would not feel so alone. Such symptoms were often thought to be uncommon with this disease, and providers would tell patients that their emotional symptoms were unrelated. This thinking seems laughable at this point. Most patients relate stories of anxiety, depressed mood, or excessive mood swings as a symptom of their illness long before diagnosis.

Many studies (but not enough) have been done on the mood disorders most common with MS. The *Journal of*

Neurovirology reported in 2000 that emotional disturbances are common in MS and consist of alterations of mood and affect. The conditions most often seen are major depressive disorder, dysthymic disorder, bipolar disorder, panic disorder, and generalized anxiety disorder. Their relationship to MS is complex, and the extent to which they are direct consequences of the disease process or psychological reactions to it remains unclear. The symptoms of mood disorders in people with MS are no different from the symptoms of mood disorders in people without MS, and respond just as well to standard treatments. These disorders result from demyelination, or damage to the myelin sheath, and are some of the most characteristic symptoms of MS. Mood and affective disturbances can cause enormous pain and suffering and lead to significant disruption of family, work, and social life. Physicians who can identify, diagnose, treat, and manage mood and affective disturbances effectively can have a tremendous impact on the quality of life for patients and families. Mood disturbances are also common with other disorders such as Lupus, Fibromyalgia, Crohn's Disease, and Rheumatoid arthritis. Any condition that is incurable, life-long, and causes uncomfortable symptoms can lead to mood disorders.

With MS in particular, a specific type of mood disorder called *Psuedobulbar Affect (PBA)* may occur. It is estimated that up to one million people suffer from this condition worldwide, and it is caused by neurological conditions such as stroke and MS. PBA can cause what is referred to as "emotional incontinence," or uncontrollable laughing or crying. These episodes can manifest themselves as inappropriate happiness or sadness, with visible signs of emotion. Patients describe these episodes almost like "seizures," coming on rapidly, and lasting for a few minutes. Most people experience several episodes per day, and this symptom can be incredibly disabling, causing patients to fear even leaving the house.

Patients may experience laughing during very sad moments, or crying during very happy times, with no real explanation. This disorder is becoming increasingly understood and recognized by providers, and there are even some new pharmacological treatments for it. These uncontrollable emotions are not related to depression or any other psychological illness. It is important to inform friends and family about the disorder if you have been diagnosed. This way, the people in your life will be prepared in case you experience an episode in front of them. In addition, it is important to be open and honest with your provider if you are experiencing this specific MS symptom. Treatment is available, and there is nothing to be ashamed of.

Some of the most difficult aspects of MS are the ever evolving, sometimes bizarre and unclear symptoms that patients experience. We often find ourselves asking, "is this MS?" It is important to understand that MS can manifest as almost any physical, emotional, or psychological symptom, depending on the specific area of the brain that has suffered damage. As we know, the brain is the "CEO" of the entire body, and controls absolutely every bodily function. We also understand that MS is capable of causing attacks and damage to every area of the brain. Individual disease courses can be so diverse, and one individual may have primarily emotional manifestations of the disease, while another may experience purely physical decline. Please do not ever feel like you are imagining your symptoms.

In essence, the conclusion is that these mood issues result either directly from physical damage to the nervous system, or from the emotional burden of these diseases.

Many patients will find this reassuring, because so often we think of psychological distress as "crazy" or "disturbed." There is a stigma in our society, and it needs to end. Avoiding the discussion about emotional symptoms with providers only delays the treatment, and the sad part is: These symptoms are entirely manageable with the proper monitoring. Psychological manifestations of chronic illness are treatable, and usually respond very well to medications.

Fatigue is another force to be reckoned with for all patients, myself included. Often times, as I sat on the couch, my life swirled around me at the speed of light. I sat, and my family moved around the house, carrying on with a normal day. Children played, my husband bustled around cleaning, picking up toys. Friends would come and go, family members chattered on the phone. Children got ready for school, a trip to the park, or horseback riding lessons. All the while, I sat. It was a feeling like no other, this inability to get up and take part in my life. The experience of being an observer, rather than an active participant, was incredibly disturbing to me. My mind wanted desperately to get up, to join in, and be there instead of on the couch. My mind urged me, "Get up! You can do it! Let's go! Don't miss out!" But my body didn't listen. My body had a mind of its own now.

MS fatigue crippled me at times, and this was not what I imagined when I was first diagnosed. I imagined that my mind would be the same, but I would lose specific functions here and there. I pictured losing the strength in an arm, for example; but retaining all of my other functions. I imagined feeling a weakened leg on occasion, maybe some blurry vision, but I would basically be the same person. I discovered, as I am sure you have, that fatigue can be the biggest crippler of all.

My life felt like a movie at certain moments. It was as if I was sitting in a theater seat, watching images on a screen. The only difference is, the scenes passing by in front of me were my life. Laughing, running, spinning, jumping children flew past me, friends called, invitations were declined. And my internal voices did battle. The mind vs. the body: The epic saga continues.

How do we cope with fatigue? Are there any good answers? Often, we ask ourselves whether we are just being lazy, or could we be clinically depressed? The answer is typically, neither! 80% of MS patients suffer from fatigue, and it isn't your average, everyday exhaustion. It is specific to MS, and incredibly debilitating. According to the National MS Society:

"In addition to these sources of fatigue, there is another kind of fatigue — referred to as lassitude — that is unique to people with MS. Researchers are beginning to outline the characteristics of this so-called "MS fatigue" that make it different from fatigue experienced by persons without MS."

- **Generally occurs on a daily basis**
- **May occur early in the morning, even after a restful night's sleep**
- **Tends to worsen as the day progresses**
- **Tends to be aggravated by heat and humidity**
- **Comes on easily and suddenly**
- **Is generally more severe than normal fatigue**
- **Is more likely to interfere with daily responsibilities**
- **MS-related fatigue does not appear to be directly correlated with either depression or the degree of physical impairment.**

What can we do to manage this fatigue? First and foremost, see your provider. Make sure you aren't missing a treatable reason for your fatigue, such as a thyroid disorder, sleep apnea, or anemia. Once other causes are ruled out, our options (as always) are quite limited. Physical therapy might be helpful. Sleep regulation is incredibly important, and should be addressed first. Stress reduction and relaxation techniques may be helpful. Avoiding extreme heat is a must, as heat may dramatically worsen fatigue. In addition, several medications are approved for fatigue management. Provigil, Nuvigil and Symmetrel are currently FDA approved for treating fatigue.

Most importantly, make sure you are taking care of yourself in all the classic ways. Adequate hydration, nutrition, and rest are essential parts of your daily routine as a patient. Avoiding excessive caffeine and alcohol, avoiding smoking, and getting as much activity as possible are effective in combatting fatigue. Though it may seem counter-intuitive, getting some degree of physical activity can actually increase your energy, even if it is the last thing on Earth you feel like doing. Getting up and off that couch and taking in some sunlight can elevate your mood.

Consider inviting friends to visit you at your home, if you don't have the strength to go visit them. Being completely honest is essential. Let your friends and family know the degree of your struggle with fatigue, and give them the opportunity to understand. We often jump to the conclusion that, "No one gets it. No one will ever understand." Maybe they *will* if you give them a chance. Educating our family and friends about our illness is our responsibility, as patients. We should offer as much advice and information as possible to those in our circle. They will likely be happy to help if they can!

So often as patients, we are left to ponder the question, "Is it just ME?" We are experiencing a tsunami of indescribable emotions, physical sensations, cognitive issues, and life-altering choices. These sensations and emotions come and go multiple times per day, along with the accompanying analysis of said sensations. A short summary of some often-asked questions I pose to myself on an almost daily basis:

1. Have I totally lost my mind?
2. Was that emotional outburst just me, or MS?

3. When will my family finally grow completely tired of this ordeal and leave me?

4. Should I change my disease-modifying medication? I don't think it's working....

5. Did I just feel a new buzzing on my leg?

6. Has my foot numbness gotten worse?

7. Is my vision worse than usual today?

8. How many sick hours do I have left at work?

9. Where did I put my.... cell phone? (This one happens about 1000 times per day. Insert any object you repeatedly have to search for here....)

10. Why can't I remember that person's name?

With this constant stream of internal reviews and questions, it is no wonder that many of us are chronically exhausted. The *experience* of having a chronic disease is the thing I found most personally disruptive, but as a health professional, I also find it interesting from a scientific perspective. After we are diagnosed, we spend hours, days, even weeks studying and reading as much information as we can get our hands on. We begin to understand the disease inside and out, from every possible angle (from a physical point of view.) We understand the immune system, the autoimmune nature of the disease, and the medications we can use to combat the accompanying symptoms. But, nowhere to we read about how to cope with the *experience.*

What about the human experience of carrying this disease burden daily? What about that? This is why making connections with other patients is an essential part of treatment. Have you felt this way? Have you felt alone with your symptoms of anger and sadness? I am here to tell you that you are anything but alone. The best therapy is to share! If you are concerned about being judged, find a forum that you feel comfortable with. Share anonymously, if you need to, but share. Talk. Exchange ideas. Keep the information flowing, and you just might be able to help another person suffering from similar issues.

Journal 10: Mood Disorders and Fatigue:

Have you had emotional disturbances and/or fatigue? What types of feelings do you experience? Do you feel sadness, anger, frustration, or anxiety? Take a moment to write about these feelings and how you experience them.

11

Identity Crisis! Finding a New Purpose and Passion After Your Career Ends

"The purpose of life is not to be happy. It is to be useful, to be honorable, to be compassionate, to have it make some difference that you have lived and lived well."
-Ralph Waldo Emerson

Like most people, you probably spent years creating and establishing your career through education and work experience. Maybe you even had one of those childhood dreams. "I always wanted to be a......."

Maybe you spent endless days of your life in college, sweating and toiling over exams, writing endless pages of term papers, and spending long nights studying. Maybe, like me, you spent thousands of dollars on tuition and books, or took out large student loans to fund your educational pursuits. Maybe you spent years giving up life experiences in lieu of education. You may have missed weddings, birthdays, holidays, and other moments in order to pursue your degree.

I spent about eight years in college, finally earning my Masters degree in 2012. Through this pursuit, I established a new identity for myself: I was a nurse practitioner. I was proud of this title, and you are probably proud of yours. We worked hard for this, right? Isn't this who we really are? What happens when your illness takes that title away from you? What if you can no longer work? We are such a career-oriented society, telling our children from an early age to go to college and "be something." One of the most common topics of discussion between kids is "What Do YOU want to be when you grow up?"

With MS, most of us will reach a day when we can no longer find the strength, the cognition, or the ability to stay employed. We might push ourselves for years beyond the point we should, hoping that things will improve and we can continue. No matter how much we hope that things would be different, we will likely end up needing to either slow down our work, or stop altogether. It is just a matter of time, but what happens then? Would I still be able to call myself a nurse? If I am not a nurse, who am I? I had almost forgotten who I was without my professional title.

When you face a career-ending crisis, try to see it as a chance to find something brand new, exhilarating, and wonderful. It isn't necessarily the tragedy you might believe it is. Change is never easy, but sometimes it is what you need, even if it isn't something you think you want.

As a child, I loved theater, singing, dancing, and books. I loved to write poetry and creative stories. I was content with these things, and at that time I was just *myself.* These are the things I began to love passionately again. This loss of "career self" led to a rediscovery of my true self, and it was wonderful! My fifth year with MS was rough for me, and I dealt with several relapses requiring treatment. During that time, I was forced to spend time away from work. I began pulling away from my professional identity, which felt like a loss at first. I actually grieved for this identity. I dreaded losing the thing I had worked so hard for, that crowning achievement that I had earned through sweat and tears. I thought I was losing my entire existence, my whole life. Slowly though, I started to think about topics I hadn't even considered for many years. I found myself reading books that weren't medical texts! I found myself writing for the joy of it, rather than writing because a term paper was due. The interesting thing is, I found myself going back to the things I loved BEFORE I was a nurse practitioner.

I started to enjoy blogging and sharing my experiences. I had time to spend with my children, and now I actually listened to them, helped with homework, and had conversations. I played board games with my kids, discussed the future, swam with them in the pool, and sat together with my family under the stars by the fire pit. I had coffee with my close friends and family, and I enjoyed the warmth of the sun, the colors of the fall landscape, the smile on my husband's face, and the beauty of it all. If I could potentially help just one patient through my writing, I felt that my life had purpose and meaning, and this would continue even if I were no longer employed. I started to understand that the *ending* I thought I was experiencing might perhaps just be a new beginning. If it weren't for my illness, I would likely be unable to experience these simple, beautiful moments. Time became precious, and my appreciation of the scarcity of it grew every day.

"Be patient... Wait... No rush...You have plenty of time..."

How many times during your life have you heard these words of wisdom being uttered by those around you?

I was always a very determined, sometimes slightly "manic" person when I had my focus set on something I wanted to do, and it may have appeared sometimes that I was rushing, hurrying, and pushing the limits. This was not really the case, however. After I was diagnosed with MS, I had a sense of urgency that I never knew before. My time was unknown, undetermined, unpredictable. Tomorrow, I may or may not have the same cognitive and physical abilities that I had today.

It is a very interesting way of life, isn't it? Living with an illness that threatens to take your functions away on a daily basis. It can be an incredible depressant, or it can motivate like nothing else. The luxury of time is something we just simply do not have. My focus eventually changed to writing, and it gave me a sense of continued purpose for many years. As long as I continued to write, I felt as though the beast would not catch me. The monster would not quite be able to overtake me. Just write...write...write...

The entre mindset shifts with a chronic illness, and time no longer seems like something that exists in an endless supply. It becomes rare, precious, priceless in our eyes, because it is a commodity that may be taken from us in an instant. How do we cope? How do we avoid being sucked into the void of depression? How do we use this awareness of the value of time to our advantage? Because the truth is, it may actually be a gift in disguise.

The awareness of time. It is the opposite of rushing through the day, hurrying from place to place. It is the antithesis of racing through daily obligations, ignorant of the beautiful things happening all around you. The awareness of time is the practice of being truly in the moment. Looking around, taking it all in. The colors, smells, sounds, and the feelings. The temperature, tastes, and the observations. This is the place we all should be, but it seems to be impossible for so many in our hurried society.

If you have found yourself out of work because of your illness, disabled, unable to spend your days at a job, you may have the opportunity to experience true awareness of time. This is a gift; one that many people will never have the opportunity to enjoy. This awareness takes practice, but give it a try. Even sitting in your own home, you may begin to notice the things around you that were taken for granted previously. If you are still working and parenting, busily raising children and trying to make ends meet, the awareness and appreciation of time is more difficult. Not impossible, however.

Your time is even more limited, rare, and scarce. You must work even harder to find that precious moment of awareness. The stress of daily life interferes with our ability to notice the simple things in life, and this is the unfortunate reality for most people. The battle to both maintain a household and family, and enjoy our lives is ongoing and difficult. If we don't work at it, it generally will not happen. Make enjoyment and awareness a priority in your life, no matter what the circumstances may be. Sometimes MS forces us to let go of the things we formerly saw as crucial, and define an entirely new set of priorities. As I let go of my career, I realized that my struggle to cling to it was a manifestation of my own perfectionistic ideals.

I was always a textbook perfectionist, but only when it came to myself. It's fine for everyone else to make mistakes, but I expected way more of myself. I was overly concerned with details, and I was my own worst critic. This is a very difficult way to live, and this way of thinking causes a great deal of pain in the end. The fact of the matter is that no one is perfect. The goal of perfection is unachievable, so attempting it is only bound to lead to heartbreak.

What we need to keep in mind as MS patients is, our family and friends do not have the same lofty expectations of us that we have for ourselves. Our friends and family love us unconditionally, and basically just want us to be *around.* I was so hard on myself sometimes. When I was invited to an event, I found myself thinking, "This is a happy occasion, and no one is going to want to deal with me and my illness. It is just baggage, and it is so depressing. I just won't even go."

Here's the thing: Those thoughts are damaging, and they are entirely untrue. What I found after years with MS is, those who cared about me wanted me to be *present,* even if I was not *perfect.* No one expects perfection, and on the contrary, many friends were so understanding, so helpful, and so supportive. Would I have ever known this had I simply stayed home in fear? Don't waste your time feeling like a burden to others, because you will end up self-defeating. You will end up stuck at home, shut in, and deprived of the happy life that you deserve.

This pursuit of perfectionism will steal your life. It will paralyze you, leaving you terrified that you aren't "good enough." This fear is real, and it is a killer. We must remain aware of it's potential to steal our happiness. Each year with MS may bring a new disability, a new deficit, or a new symptom. We have to remain in a state of constant evolution, changing our approach to life, changing how we perform our daily tasks. Included with this, we need to change our self-image. From day to day, our external and internal image may be entirely different. We may need a cane on Monday, but by Wednesday, we are walking just fine with no assistance. With those changes, we must learn how to change our perception of ourselves. Do not allow any symptom, any deficit, or any disability to define who you are, or stop you from attaining your goals. Remember, the goal is to be *present not perfect.*

Your illness does not define you, but it is a part of your reality. The people in your life who truly care about you will not leave your life simply because of illness. Granted, you may lose a few "friends" you had before your illness, those who cannot handle the issue and would rather leave your life. The truth is, it is their loss. It is about them, and not you. It is not your business what other people think of you, as they say.

Try not to allow worry, perfectionism, or self-consciousness to drive your life. You take the wheel, instead. Don't miss out on opportunities to experience and enjoy your life simply because of your illness. The people around you who truly love will not mind if you carry along your "baggage," and they may even offer to help you carry it once in a while.

Try to have faith that those around you will understand that you have flaws, you have an illness that is incurable, and you are doing your very best to cope with it. I would venture to guess that you would be pleasantly surprised by the outcome. By letting go of the attempts at perfection and being brave enough to show our flaws, we find real love. We find out who will be there, no matter what. And that is a beautiful discovery.

Human beings crave a purpose. For many people, the career is the primary source of purpose and meaning. When that career fades, the key is to find your passion. Do you love to read, sing, dance, write, draw, listen to music, or volunteer for charities? Find something that drives you, excites you, and makes you feel fulfilled. You are more than that title you earned in school; you are unique, capable, and valuable even after employment ends. Even more importantly, you are an essential part of your family's lives, and they want you around no matter how severe your symptoms are. Just being present for your children and family is enough.

Journal 11: Identity and Awareness:

Who were you as a young child? What did you enjoy doing before you had a career? What is your passion, what drives you? Do you stop to enjoy the "little things" when you can? What have you noticed that you find particularly beautiful?

12

Loss of Independence and Grief: Ghosts of the Past

"The most beautiful people I've known are those who have known trials, have known struggles, have known loss, and have found their way out of the depths."
-Elisabeth Kubler-Ross

The process of letting go of our former selves is a long and difficult one, much like grieving, with distinct stages. I believe we need to allow ourselves time to grieve the loss of the person we always thought we would be. After all, this is a great loss. We lose our identities, and we naturally need to recover.

In her landmark work, *On Death and Dying*, Elizabeth Kubler-Ross described grief as having the following stages: Denial, Anger, Bargaining, Depression, and Acceptance. In her model, Kubler-Ross describes each of these stages as distinct. Each stage can last for days, weeks, months, or even years. I can say that I felt definite denial and anger stages in my five years with MS. Acceptance: I am not there yet. I am working on it, but I am not there. We must allow ourselves time to pass through each phase on our own terms. No one should ever tell you that you should be "over it" by now, because it is no one else's decision or process, it is yours.

Patients with chronic illnesses don't just experience one loss, but many evolving losses. This is the essence of the difficulty of the disease. One loss can be grieved and managed, but daily, incremental, changeable losses are much harder to recover from. Grief becomes not just one distinct process, but a series of processes that are unending for those coping with an illness. This continued loss of function, cognition, and identity are the reason they can be such difficult diseases to live with *forever.* The concept of an incurable, life long illness is a difficult thing to accept, mainly because "forever" is an idea that does not apply to many situations in most lives. Chronic illness is like receiving a brand, tattoo, or lifetime label. It will never go away, and we each need to come to terms with this.

We must remain aware of the fact that though every individual may not have a chronic illness, every human being faces difficulties in life. No one escapes with a perfect, pain free existence. Everyone has challenges that are unique. Some are struggling with financial troubles and poverty, some are consumed with emotional and psychological difficulties, and others are fighting physical ailments. Though these issues may vary from person to person, we are all connected as human beings through these life battles. Not everyone you know may have an illness, but remember that everyone you know is fighting a battle that you may know nothing about. No one has a perfect life, even if they don't carry the burden of disease.

I want you to know that if you have days when you feel the need to process your grief, do not feel guilty. You may have days where you don't want to be cheered up, told to "stay strong" and fight. Some days are made for fighting, and some are made for processing your grief; and it is normal and healthy to do so. It can be very difficult to communicate this fact to our loved ones, who only aim to cheer us up. We may have moments that cause us to want to be alone, to process our grief. Our loved ones may not understand, and may even find this concerning. It is important to communicate that processing is an essential part of grief.

Loss of independence causes more grief, and the losses are continuous at times. Many patients may start out as fiercely independent people, but may find that they need help here and there due to illness. This can be incredibly difficult for most patients, especially those who are young and not accustomed to asking for help. I found that my own losses of independence were a source of great distress, and it was difficult for me to accept help from others.

A commonly heard phrase now echoed throughout my house: "Honey, can you open this jar for me?" I have always been an extremely independent, (some may say stubborn) individual. I detested feeling dependent on others, especially my close friends and family. In fact, one of the first thoughts I had after my MS diagnosis was: "*I refuse to be someone's burden!*"

There are little things that happened each day, my inability to open a jar, my inability to drive at night, my fatigue in the afternoons. Then, there were larger issues such as my inability to earn a living the way I used to, the missed children's football and soccer games due to heat and flares, and the emotional impact this illness had on my husband and children. How do you cope with this loss of independence? It is almost inevitable that this diagnosis goes hand in hand with increased dependence on others.

The chronically ill patients I met in the last few years are just like me. Most of us are very strong, stubborn, independent individuals who feel just as I do. I found myself feeling guilty every time I had to ask for help. Apparently, this was my life lesson, my challenge, and my major life obstacle to overcome. Life seems to continue to present tests and challenges until we learn them thoroughly, and dependence on others was a major obstacle in my own life.

As I examined my motivations and feelings more closely, I realized that a lot of these feelings were purely my ego. I gained self-esteem from being independent, and I always had. I had a constant little voice in my mind throughout my life asking "would you be okay if you were on your own completely? If you lost everyone you know?" My answer was always a resounding: "YES!" However, now I realize that this was not a healthy mindset. Now, I had much to lose.

In the past, I mistakenly saw my lack of dependence as strength. I thought that because I had nothing to lose, I was untouchable emotionally. No one could ever hurt me if

I did not care that much; I needed nothing from anyone, and I liked it that way. I protected and shielded myself from harm by pretending I was completely independent. I thought this was the way I wanted to live, the safe way to get through life. Boy, was I wrong. My conclusion became much different after living with MS, and I now realized that I needed to feel supported by others. It is a basic human need.

The question then, is: How do you do this? How do you accept your small (or large) losses of independence? My answer is that your *loss* may actually be your *gain*.

When you ask for help you:

1. Show that you are trusting of another human being.

2. Show that you are in need at the moment, but not forever.

3. Develop a bond with another human being.

4. Form the foundation of a long, connected relationship.

5. Create an opportunity to help someone else in the near future.

How great would that feel? To know without a doubt that your friend/spouse/caregiver/family member will always be there for you, no matter what? This is what I gained when I lost. I may have needed help opening my next jar, but I had a lifelong bond with my spouse that was reinforced each time I needed a hand. Do not mistake needing help for weakness, or independence for power. Resilience comes from building strong relationships with those closest to you. This is where our true strength lies.

Many MS patients experience grief after diagnosis, and grief is a process that our bodies use to respond to loss. It is a necessary process, one that cannot be sped up or manipulated to fit our needs. We need to experience each stage of grief as it comes, in order to fully recover. Do not rush through your grief, but rather allow it guide you through each of the distinct stages you may experience.

Kubler-Ross Grief Stages Applied to MS

1. Denial: The individual cannot completely face the diagnosis, and pushes the reality out of view. Creates a

false "reality," ignoring the actual loss until they are better able to face it.

2.   Anger: This is the "Why me?" phase. The patient feels rage, sadness, and anger about the situation. Questions why something so terrible would happen to THEM?

3.   Bargaining: The patient begins to slightly accept the diagnosis, but still cannot completely cope. Thinks, "Maybe the doctors were wrong? Maybe the diagnosis is incorrect?"

4.   Depression: When reality finally sinks in. The patient understands that the diagnosis is indeed correct, and becomes extremely despondent about it. Crying, hiding at home, not participating in usual activities.

5.   Acceptance: The patient finally accepts the diagnosis. They realize that nothing can be done to change it, and now they need to start living in spite of

it. The patient experiences a calm, retrospective view. "It's going to be ok. I can fight this."

These phases can come in any order, and can last for any period of time. This grieving process is necessary in order for the patient to move on, accept the diagnosis, and start to prepare for a life with illness. Patients may not be able to accurately explain this process to friends and family, and many may not understand that they are experiencing a normal grief reaction. It is imperative that caregivers and friends understand that this process is absolutely essential to the patient's well-being. Patients need to grieve in order to recover from the shock of the diagnosis, and start a life beyond illness. Sometimes, making connections with other MS patients and sharing experiences is a wonderful way to assist in the grieving process.

As I experienced my grief, I found myself in awe of the power of technology. I formed connections with MS patients worldwide, and using the power of the internet, I found others who were experiencing exactly the same thing that I was. I felt so fortunate to live in this time, because with an illness like MS, feeling understood and supported is absolutely essential. For those who have no friends and family with MS, the virtual support system found online can be life saving. There is nothing more dangerous than feeling isolated, alone, and misunderstood. Once we begin to feel alone, we start to sink into dark places and depression.

Connections help us reach up out of that darkness into the light again. For those who feel uncomfortable attending in-person support groups, MS related online groups, chats, and conversations could be just as effective. The outpouring of support I received from virtual support systems reassured me that people around the world were listening, and hopefully feeling a bit better by reading these words I typed. Do you find yourself thinking, "I must be the only one feeling this way?" I often had those thoughts. I often thought that I must be the only one on the planet who has ever reacted in this way. It only took me about 10 seconds in my virtual "support groups" to realize that I was never the only one.

My grandmother had MS during the 1950s. My mother explained to me that in that time, no one discussed MS. It was a family secret, something that was not mentioned in public. Can you imagine if you were made to feel by society that MS was shameful? It must have been so difficult to suffer from MS in previous generations, before a definite understanding of the disease.

MS researchers are tirelessly working on new, novel treatments for our illness. As we try our best to manage the disease and cope with current treatment options, they continue to work, study, learn, and develop new treatment strategies. I feel so reassured when I read about new studies, new generations of researchers and scientists devoting entire careers to the eradication of this disease. Do not underestimate the power of basic human communication when managing your illness. Sometimes, we are powerless over the physical symptoms we experience with MS, but we are always in control of the way we *react.*

"When we meet real tragedy in life, we can react in two ways - either by losing hope and falling into self-destructive habits, or by using the challenge to find our inner strength." - Dalai Lama

I like to think of MS as a challenge to improve the person I was before, to find new strength, and to develop a stronger mind. If we are never challenged, we can never grow. I know that sometimes, we don't want to hear the "cheerleading," the inspirational quotes, and the over-the-top positivity. However, sometimes those things are exactly what we need. If all else fails, and you still feel down and depressed, try this: Try to support and cheer another MS patient; if not in person, then online. Try to provide the support and positivity that you would like to have. Try to pull another patient up from the depths of sadness, and you might actually feel energized, renewed, and valuable. Your experience is very likely to be incredibly helpful to another struggling patient. Human connections are the key, and sometimes a computer/phone/tablet is the only tool required. Grief is a process, and we must allow ourselves the time to leave behind our former identities, while creating new and beautiful lives.

Journal 12: Loss and Grief:

What things you have lost that bother you the most? Have you grieved for lost abilities, jobs, or friends? Have you processed these losses? Do you feel more comfortable asking for help than you did previously? How did YOU learn to ask for help?

13

Pain and Substance Abuse

"Numbing the pain will only make it worse when you finally feel it." –JK Rowling

I stumbled, having consumed my second drink of the evening, a vodka and diet coke. It was my "go-to" drink, one that I poured with regularity in the evening, thinking nothing of it. I felt the warm, calm tingling of alcohol induced relaxation fall from my shoulders to my ankles. I made my way toward my medicine cabinet. My evening medications were due, the anxiety meds, the pain meds, the sleep meds. I nearly choked on one as I swallowed, and I looked around the bathroom. Is this really what my life has become? I was alone. My husband was at work, and my children were in bed. Was this the way I wanted to live? This was a moment that stands out in my memory. I was using too many medications, and relying too heavily on them as a crutch. It dulled my pain, helped ease my anxiety, and made life seem better. But, in my heart, I knew that I could not continue in this manner.

My daily pain was a burden, a weight on my shoulders. I carried it through every day, and every sleepless night. I had severe extremity, hip, lower back and facial pain. I had never experienced pain like this in my entire life, and it caused me to feel extremely depressed about my future. As a nurse practitioner, I dealt with chronic pain patients often, and frankly, they got a bad rap. Many were seen as "drug seekers," merely trying to feed their opiate addictions through false complaints of pain. I developed a hardened attitude toward chronic pain patients, whispered to other health providers, looked disparagingly on those who returned frequently for unproven pain. Suddenly, I realized I was one of them now.

Managing the symptoms of MS is the most important focus for each of us. Pain can be one of the most vexing symptoms for many patients, and pain can seriously diminish quality of life. Pain comes in two forms, acute and chronic, and the body has very different mechanisms in place for coping with each. There is a striking difference between pain that is acute in nature (sudden injury/fracture/laceration severe headache,) and pain that is chronic (daily, ongoing, unchanging, long-term.) The body has mechanisms in place to cope with sudden, severe pain, with responses mimicking the "flight or flight" response. The body responds with adrenaline, increased heart rate and blood pressure, and natural pain response chemicals (endorphins) that help to ease the pain a bit. The body mounts an all-out response to sudden illness and pain, and is well equipped to cope with these periodic occurrences.

How does the body cope with pain that is chronic? Pain that is daily, ongoing, never relenting, and does not stop? What about pain that goes on for weeks, months, or years? As it turns out, the body isn't very good at coping with this type of pain, the pain that many experience with multiple sclerosis. Chronic pain can become one of the most physically and psychologically difficult symptoms, and should never be ignored or brushed off by providers.

MS pain can be episodic, experienced only during a relapse, or it can be a daily battle for many patients, as well as a nightly one, causing insomnia. Pain can result from inappropriate nerve response to the damage caused by MS, or it can result from spasticity (muscle spasm,) also a product of damaged nerves. Regardless of the type, most

MS patients will cope with chronic pain at some point. Varying types of pain tend to affect MS patients, but the most common include:

- **Trigeminal neuralgia** — This is a sharp, excruciating pain affecting the face, usually on one side. This can often be extremely debilitating, and is often mistaken for dental pain. This syndrome can occur without MS, but it is far more common in MS patients than the general population. (At one time called "the suicide disease" because so many patients ended their lives after suffering from the intense pain.)

- **Burning pain in arms and legs**— Touch sensitivity, alterations in skin sensation, and a deep, burning pain may occur in MS patients. This pain is caused by demyelination and damage to nerves. Pain can be located just about anywhere, but the limbs are the most common location.

- **L'Hermette's sign and other neck pain** —Some patients experience a sharp electrical jolt when the chin is brought down to the chest. Other, inexplicable neck and back pain can occur, including spasm.

- **Joint pain related to steroids**— Some patients develop avascular necrosis, or reduction in blood flow to hip and shoulder joints due to lifelong steroid use. X-ray and MRI are used to evaluate joint damage. Surgery may be necessary for this issue. If you have ongoing joint pain in one particular location, it is important to have it evaluated.

Unfortunately, we don't have a lot of great medications to choose from for chronic pain. There are medications like gabapentin (Neurontin) and Lyrica that may help calm nerve pain. There are anti-spasmotic drugs such as Baclofen or Zanaflex that can calm spasticity. These may take the edge off, but many patients still experience daily pain.

Opiate medications such as Vicodin and Norco (hydrocodone) are not good answers for chronic types of pain, because they can lead to dependence. These medications are designed only for short term, acute pain types. Many chronic pain patients end up needing more and more opiate medications, eventually leading to severe dependency and addiction issues.

My opinion as a healthcare provider is, opiates should never be started for MS related chronic pain because these medications are a *dead-end road*. They only lead to more problems. Do we *really* need more problems? I had several close friends who became dependent on opiate medications, and I saw first hand the devastating consequences of prescription drug abuse while working in healthcare. It is better to never even consider these medications for pain management if you don't absolutely have to. As always, follow the advice of your pain specialist or neurologist.

Medication and traditional treatment aside, how does the mind *cope* with this pain on a daily basis? I felt pain on a daily basis for several years, and it was unrelenting. I never appreciated how life-altering chronic pain can become, as I spent the first three years after diagnosis pain-free. I felt so fortunate at that time, but soon began to experience muscle spasm, leaving me feeling like I had just run a marathon every single day. The muscle pain was so intense that I could not walk on some days. I had neck and shoulder pain that shot from my neck, down to the shoulder, clavicle, and down my arm. I also began to experience facial pain, a severe type of dental pain on one side that was eventually diagnosed as trigeminal neuralgia.

My neurologist was excellent, helping me find the right "cocktail" of medications for pain, including gabapentin three times daily, Tegretol (an anti-seizure drug that is indicated for trigeminal neuralgia), and Baclofen daily for spasm. I had good days and bad days, but on many days I felt fairly severe pain by the end of the day. Healthy people often ask, "What is the worst pain that a human being can experience? Is it childbirth? Kidney stones? Fractures?" These examples of acute pain may indeed be classified as the most intense types, but they are time limited. Childbirth doesn't go on forever. Kidney stones eventually pass, and fractures heal. With chronic types of pain, there is no end in sight.

One of the problems that go hand-in-hand with chronic pain is substance abuse. It is a dangerous, tempting road for those who cope with daily pain. The temptation to ease pain by taking a drink is very real; unfortunately, alcohol does ease the pain, but as we know, it is no solution. It is another dead-end road. I experienced the euphoric relief that alcohol gave me, but I had to fight the urge to have another, and another tomorrow, and another the next day. It is not the answer. So, what IS the answer?

A National Institute of Health study notes: "Substance abuse may be present in 19% of MS patients and contribute to high rates of depression. There may be greater risk of harm due to substance abuse in people with MS because of the potential magnification of motor and cognitive impairments. Comprehensive MS care should include substance abuse screening and advice to cut down or abstain from use" (NIH, 2014.)

In essence, the effects of alcohol and drugs on MS patients are amplified, causing existing MS deficits like balance problems and weakness to become even more severe. Though the immediate pain relief these substances provide us might be tempting, we must see these substances as a poor solution. Increased balance issues and weakness while consuming alcohol can potentially lead to falls and other injuries. We must find solutions that we can use for a lifetime; solutions that can be maintained daily, for the rest of our lives, safely and effectively.

Alternative treatments such as biofeedback, acupuncture, massage, meditation, and yoga have been studied and found to show potential for the treatment of chronic pain for some patients. Studies are ongoing regarding the use of medical marijuana for MS pain and spasticity, and initial findings look hopeful. Medical marijuana may indeed be effective for these specific symptoms, but not for much else. However, if it indeed gives pain relief to MS patients, thereby avoiding the more dangerous drugs such as opiates, then it is a positive option. More testing needs to be done, but it looks promising. The key is to find *your* magic combination. Try not to make assumptions about whether or not a treatment might work for you; give it a try if you get the okay from your provider.

Alternative therapies, fad diets, and supplements provide new dilemmas for patients and providers alike. The way in which prescription treatments are created is through a scientific, data-oriented study model. This model requires years and years of study, beginning in the lab, progressing to animal studies, then to human trials over a great deal of time. The twelve disease-modifying drugs we currently have in our arsenal in 2015 were developed during a course of strenuous scientific research, with the top minds in the world putting tremendous effort into the various phases of testing. They were approved by the FDA, and found to be effective over a long period of time.

Other than our 12 disease modifying drugs, we have no other information about effective MS treatments at this point in time. Studies are always ongoing, and alternative treatments may prove themselves over the course of time. Buyer and patient beware: Your provider knows best. Do your research. Do not ever try an alternative treatment unless you get the okay from your neurologist or other treating provider. There are unlimited numbers of scam artists just waiting to prey on defenseless MS patients and our desperation for a cure.

HMOs and insurers of all types focus on *reducing costs and using less treatment* rather than more treatment. They aim to spend less money on medication for patients, rather than more. Insurers would, in a heartbeat- recommend dietary changes over the current $50,000-$60,000 per year expense of MS drugs if these diets were proven. Think of the cost savings for all HMOs! Why would they ever pay for medication when a simple diet change would do the trick? The answer is: They would not. The problem is, there is no data to show these diets work.

Contrary to the claims of "fad diets" advertising to MS patients, there is no known diet that has ever been proven to treat MS at this time. Unfortunately, these diets have only led to frustration for many patients who have tried them, hoping for tremendous improvement. The concept that diet can reduce or even "cure" MS symptoms is simply incorrect from a scientific standpoint at this point in time. There are anecdotal tales of individual patients improving after trying certain dietary changes, but this has simply not been proven in clinical trials. This way of thinking causes MS patients who are progressing to feel that they are at fault. "If only you had eaten the right things you would be fine," is an attitude that is damaging and depressing. It inflicts harm on patients who have tried and failed with dietary changes. Perhaps down the road, through scientific study, this viewpoint may change.

The trouble with supplements or alternative therapies sold as "treatments," is that these therapies have not ever been proven either. If they had, why would we not be using them? Some will argue that "Big Pharma" is in charge, manipulating and controlling these drugs, milking MS patients for lifetimes of money in exchange for drugs. This may be partially true, but this is the unfortunate system we have in place. Big Pharma may indeed be making a killing on MS drugs, but that does not discount their efficacy. These drugs do indeed work, and it has been proven over and over.

In addition, every patient should be aware that supplements are a potentially dangerous road. The entire supplement industry is unregulated, untested, and unproven. They do not have to follow the rigorous guidelines that FDA approved prescription drugs follow. Anyone can literally hang a shingle, open a shop, and sell "dietary supplements" that claim to do all sorts of wonderful things. These are not proven, effective treatments, no matter what anyone claims. The other danger is financial: These products are, at the very least- a waste of money. At the very worst, they may be outright dangerous. Who knows? They *have not been tested.*

This is not to say that a healthy, well-balanced diet, daily exercise, and a generally healthy lifestyle is unwise. Following the basic guidelines for living a healthy life is good advice for anyone, not just MS patients. All of us would feel better getting regular physical activity, avoiding high fat, high sugar diets, and avoiding smoking, alcohol, and illicit drugs. These basic lifestyle changes are beneficial, but they certainly won't cure your MS.

If you would like more information on the American Academy of Neurology's statement on Alternative therapies, go to: https://www.aan.com/Guidelines/Home/GetGuidelineCon tent/644.

Chronic pain and other symptoms of MS have no specific cure, and only a handful of treatment modalities. Many patients often find nothing but disappointment at the doctor's office when they are told, "There is nothing more we can do for this symptom."

"Did you call your Doctor?" How many times have you been asked this question? Isn't it just a natural part of the experience? We are so trained to immediately assume that something can, or should be done for every physical ailment. The truth is, there isn't always an answer, there isn't always a quick fix, and in the case of most chronic illnesses, there isn't always a cure.

When a new symptom emerged, I often heard my loved ones ask me to immediately run to the phone, and let my neurologist know. I had been on a disease modifying medication for the entire course of my five years with MS, and I had been treated for dozens of relapses in that time. My average yearly relapse rate was about 6-7 per year, which is quite a lot for RRMS. Most of the time, I was treated with steroids such as Prednisone and Solu-Medrol for each relapse, and then life carried on.

The next question I usually got after the "Doctor" one was: "Did the steroids help? Are you feeling better?" The answer was typically, no. Steroids do take effect almost immediately, but it can take days, weeks, months, or years for symptoms to resolve; or they may never go away. The typical expectation is that the Doctor fixes all, and that the treatment is immediately effective. This is something that has become an underlying expectation in our society. Unfortunately, patients learn quickly that our options for treatment, as well as the successful outcomes of such treatment, are less than awe-inspiring.

Our selection of disease modifying therapies has skyrocketed from a whopping ZERO in 1992, to twelve today. Some of these are even oral drugs, not the injectable drugs we were literally "stuck with" for so many years. Having these options is something I am very grateful for, and I do not take this for granted. The frustration lies in the fact that these therapies are not cures. They are treatments, and none are perfect. They reduce annual relapse rates by varying percentages, and they lower the number of lesions visible on MRI to varying degrees. Most patients will tell you, however, that these are not perfect fixes. When we do have a relapse, we are left with steroids as our go-to medications, and we all know what a drag they can be.

As patients, we learn that running to the doctor's office often won't get us anywhere. We are often left with no clear answers, no clear options, and a variety of possible treatment modalities that may or may not help. We begin to run our own care after a few years. We know when we need steroids, when our medications are no longer doing the trick, and when to notify the doctor. We learn to evaluate and assess our bodies in a way that healthy people never do. We learn how much heat we can tolerate, how much exertion we can handle, and how much stress we can endure. We are the masters of our own bodies. The assessment is ongoing, and we never stop scanning for potential new symptoms.

The simplest of questions are often left unanswered. "Am I having a relapse?" The answer is that no one can really tell you for sure. There are guidelines; such as *new or worsening symptoms lasting 1 day or longer, separated from the last episode by 30 days or more* constitutes "relapse," but there is no diagnostic test. MRI often does not correlate with physical clinical symptoms. An MRI can look horrendous, while a patient feels fine; likewise, an MRI can look perfect while a patient feels awful. MRI is great for diagnosing MS, but after that the benefits are questionable.

Individual neurologists tend to have very different treatment modalities, including preferred drug choices, relapse treatment options, and frequency of MRIs. Some neurologists tend to be very "bare bones," meaning that they use minimal MRIs, are hesitant to treat every symptom that arises, and are unlikely to treat relapses unless they are very severe. Others might be more eager to treat each and every new symptom with steroids, order new MRI every 6 months, and use every possible resource for management of the illness. The key is to find a neurologist who takes you seriously, listens when you need them to, and communicates openly. Accessibility to care is another important factor, because relapse can occur on any given day of the year. You need to be able to contact your provider easily and quickly if needed.

MS is a difficult disease to live with for a myriad of reasons, but frustration at the doctor's office can be one of the biggest irritants. We have a serious, terrifyingly unpredictable disease that cannot always be helped by medicine. Treatments are imperfect, fraught with side effects, and incredibly expensive. All we can do is hold on and remain hopeful that our inevitable cure is just around the corner, and remember that there are brilliant research scientists committing lifetimes to finding it.

Pain specialists are found worldwide, and the treatment of chronic pain conditions such as MS is a medical subspecialty. Certain physicians specialize in the management of chronic pain, and it is important for MS patients to connect with a specialist such as this. You cannot manage your pain without help. For those like me who don't like to ask for help, you must. For those who feel that they can manage this type of pain without treatment, please reach out. No one should suffer daily from any pain unnecessarily, and treatment can improve your life dramatically. Don't waste one day suffering, when there is a world out there for you to experience.

Journal 13: Pain and Substance Abuse:

Have you coped with MS related pain? Have you had issues with alcohol or other drugs? How have you experienced pain, and what have you done to seek help? Have you found relief from anything specific?

PART THREE:
METAMORPHOSIS

14

Pursuit of Hardship: Be Your Own Hero

"A hero is an ordinary individual who finds the strength to persevere and endure in spite of overwhelming obstacles."-Christopher Reeve

Think of all the greats.

The individuals we view as being the geniuses of our time, authors, poets, painters, scientists, performers, spiritual leaders, Nobel Prize winners, and the humanitarians of the world. What makes them so incredibly gifted? I cannot say for certain, but one common thread I have observed is that many have coped with difficulties and life challenges.

Some of these people struggled with physical and mental illness, some with tragic life experiences and others with broken hearts. Some endured a horrible childhood, and others carried the burden of abuse and poverty. Such struggles and challenges could have easily steered these individuals in the wrong direction. They could have become criminals, outsiders, anti-social human beings, angry at the world and life in general. Wouldn't you have predicted that they would end up abject failures?

Astonishingly, in nearly every case the opposite is true. These individuals became the ultimate success stories of the human race. What that means to me is that there is hope. What this lesson teaches me is that my own personal challenges might actually be my biggest blessings in disguise. I know what you are thinking. "Is she serious? I should see MS (or whatever your particular life challenges are) as a gift?"

Bear with me.....

I had what most people would call an idyllic childhood. I was raised by two loving parents, and I was their only child. My parents provided me with everything a child could possibly want or need. My parents did this intentionally, because they both had less than perfect childhoods. As wonderful as this was for me, I craved more. I recall actually *wanting* to experience some traumatic events. I wanted to escape my protective childhood bubble and really get into the trenches. There is something so interesting about the experience of hardship. I firmly believe that challenges are the key to growth and the development of strength.

For me, the pursuit of hardship began with a career in emergency medical care at the age of 19, as an EMT on an advanced life support ambulance. I was like a deer in the headlights. I remember those horribly brutal calls like they happened yesterday, even though it was 20 years ago now. The first calls involving death, violence, horrific auto accidents, and tragic illness are burned into my memory. I didn't run away.

I actually found myself becoming an "adrenaline junkie." Instead of being scared away, I decided to continue and become an emergency department registered nurse at the age of 26. There is something powerful and addictive about being on edge and ready for anything all the time. I craved the teamwork, the ego boost and the indescribable feeling of saving someone from the brink of death.

I didn't really have any personal hardship, I only dealt with the hardship of others for a living. When I went home, my life was great, but I found myself picking up extra shifts at the ER just to experience some more. I *loved* being there. I met and fell in love with my husband there. The team experience of working together with excellent nurses and physicians in the ER is indescribable. Dealing with death as the "enemy" on a daily basis creates strong bonds among staff members, and there is nothing like it. Most of us could never imagine doing anything else with our lives, and felt that this was truly our calling. Along with this career path comes a sensation that we were untouchable. We were the healers, the saviors, and never the patients. We were invincible, so we thought.

In 2009, when I was diagnosed with multiple sclerosis, I no longer needed to pursue that adrenaline rush. I no longer needed to see other people's struggles to feel alive. I no longer needed to provide constant care for others in distress. It was a shocking shift in thinking, and now I was the one who finally needed help. The experience of lying in one of my own department ER beds and being tended to by nurses and physicians I worked side by side with was life changing, and now I was the one who needed the assistance. I had my first real-life *hardship.*

"Multiple Sclerosis."

What did you think when you first heard those words from the mouth of your Physician? Did pictures flash through your mind, of disability, decline, and dependence? What powerful words they are. They carry with them so many terrifying thoughts, feelings, and images. With the diagnosis comes a mask, of sorts.

This mask is one that we immediately begin to wear on day one of diagnosis. This is our "MS mask," the one that we wear to depict our disease. This is almost the equivalent of a crown being placed on the head of a new leader, except our mask isn't a positive one. It comes with fear, powerlessness, inability, and weakness. This mask tells the world that we are MS patients, we are no longer "normal," no longer "healthy," and we no longer fit in. This mask is a public one; and it is worn at all times. No matter how hard we pull and tug on it, it won't budge. This mask is a permanent one. It can never be removed, never hidden, never forgotten. Forever. On our good days, we try to hide it. We push it from our minds, we carry on with our normal activities, and we pretend it doesn't exist. However, when we least expect it, we remember... It is still there. It always will be.

How do we carry on and continue like this? How do we develop new relationships, meet the love of our lives, get married, have children, maintain a career and friendships, buy homes, and celebrate holidays all while wearing this mask? Won't it stop us from living our lives?

Won't it prevent us from doing all of the wonderful things that people long to do during life? The answer is, no.

This mask, though it's presence is permanent, has no power to control your life. This diagnosis, though it is incurable, has no ability to prevent you from achieving the goals you have set for yourself. "Normal" is *irrelevant.* It is meaningless. You do not have to be "normal" in order to live a wonderful, fulfilling life. What is normal, anyway? Normal is a concept that does not truly exist. Every single life is fraught with various difficulties, and yours just happens to be illness. This illness has no power over your life unless you give your power away. Though your physical body may be weakened at times, your mind is still your own, and you have ultimate control over that, no matter what.

MS is a lifelong struggle, a constant load of baggage that you carry around from the moment you are diagnosed. You basically have to make the choice every single day to get up, carry on, and never give in. This is a disease that requires a mantra of "I will not give in today." At any moment, if I let up, I knew the illness would catch up to me, like running from a terrifying monster in a nightmare. The sense I got was that the minute I stopped fighting this beast, it would overtake me.

Why do human beings seem to thrive under extreme conditions? Why don't we just curl up into a fetal position and give up? We are resilient and defiant. These qualities make us ultimately capable of surviving and thriving under the worst of circumstances. Difficult life events challenge our inner strength, and this process has produced some of the most incredible human beings on Earth. Hardship may push individuals to the brink of surrender, but over and over again, human beings choose to get up, stay strong, and fight. We all come from a long line of survivors! Otherwise we wouldn't be here, right?

When we receive our diagnosis of MS, most of us experience an intense identity crisis. MS causes us to re-evaluate our entire self image and re-assess our lives. Most of us immediately associate our diagnosis with disability and decline, imagining ourselves in wheelchairs or bedridden. As we now know, this is not always the case. We may live for years, decades, or even our entire lives without ever becoming severely disabled, but we have no way to predict our disease course. The problem with MS is the vast difference between individual disease processes.

One individual may become incredibly, severely disabled, and others may have minimal symptoms. The unpredictability of this illness causes an internal struggle.

I had a tendency to cripple myself emotionally with a fatalistic outlook. I found myself sinking into thoughts such as "I am ill, I am heading for complete disability, I am using a cane now, what will I be like next year? I might as well quit." I could truly be my own worst enemy, and began to recognize this self-defeating behavior. No matter how severe our disability, we may inadvertently make things seem worse than they actually are.

I call this behavior "Self-Disabling." The disease may cause physical symptoms, but my negative self-talk can be even more of a challenge. I find that I must constantly challenge the voices in my mind, the ones that tell me I am *a neurological patient with an incurable, disabling illness.* These terms, those such as "disabling", "incurable", and "progressive," can really do some damage psychologically to MS patients. Those words conjure terrifying images and strike fear into each of us. This place of fear and dread is the dark place we must avoid being trapped in. This dark place is not where we need to be. This dark place is not reality, it is a location that exists only in our minds, and we cannot allow ourselves to be stuck there.

This fear and dread caused me to often think, "Why doesn't this disease just do it's damage and be done already?" It is the slow, subtle, fluctuating nature of MS that pushes us to the brink of insanity. Most people suffer from RRMS, or relapsing remitting multiple sclerosis. This particular form of MS can be marked with severe relapses, followed by periods of almost complete remission. The time frames of each are unknown, and very individualized. The nature of this particular form of MS is unpredictability, and it is what makes it so difficult to live with. One of the first things I recall hearing my neurologist describe to me was "MS is typically *slow.*" The slow nature of the illness causes us to put ourselves in a place of illness and disability, even if we aren't truly there at the present moment.

If an individual suffers a traumatic accident, losing a limb or suffering from paralysis, this is a sudden loss of function. This individual is left to recover from the injury, knowing exactly from the first moment what the new limitations will be. For example, if the left arm is no longer useful, the individual learns to compensate with the other arm. Following the injury, there is only recovery to look forward to, and if not recovery, then adaptation to the new disability. With MS, the loss of function is fluctuating and changeable. One day, we may have to learn to live without the use of our right hand. However, we may regain this function down the road, or we may not. We can try to strengthen the use of our left hand to compensate, but then again, we may lose the function of the left hand next. I learned to cope with drop foot of my left foot by being fitted for a brace. This helped tremendously, until I lost strength in my right leg a few months later.

The unbearable unpredictability of MS is the aspect that pushes us to the edge psychologically. This unpredictable beast is the cause of the negative self-talk and fear we all live with daily. How do we rise above this place of fear and dread? How do we live a lifetime with a dangerous, unpredictable enemy living right within us? MS certainly presents a great challenge to each of us, but we need to be so grateful for the many new treatments available, and the ongoing research. We live in a time of hope and promise, as far as MS goes. We are fortunate.

Let's consider how far we have come in the battle against multiple sclerosis, from a historical perspective.

Tracing back to the middle ages, we see descriptions of patients who likely had MS. There are written logs from this era describing neurological conditions with numbness, weakness, and paralysis in otherwise young and healthy individuals. Of course, at that time there was no definitive diagnosis, and obviously no treatments.

1838: The earliest medical drawings and descriptions show patterns of illness that we now recognize as MS. The name of the illness had not been described as of yet, but physicians were making astute observations about this illness.

1868: Dr. Jean-Martin Charcot from the University of Paris (later termed the "father of neurology,") described a female patient with MS symptoms. She had slurred speech, visual problems, and tremor/weakness. After her death, she was determined to have multiple scarred areas of the brain, or plaques. We now recognize this as MS. Dr. Charcot could not determine the cause, and was unable to create any effective treatment for these patients. He tried injections of gold and silver, and the use of several poisons (these were common treatments at the time,) for these patients with no effect!

1873: MS was recognized in England by Dr. Walter Moxon, and in the United States by Dr. Edward Seguin in 1878.

1906: The Nobel Prize for Medicine was awarded to Dr. Camillo Golgi and Dr. Santiago Ramon y Cajal . These physicians were able to finally observe individual nerve cells under a microscope and see the specific damage caused by MS.

1916: Dr. James Dawson at the University of Edinburgh described that myelin was the target of MS attacks, and observed the inflammation in the brain leading to damage.

1940: The animal model of MS (EAE) was discovered, and this led to the ability to study treatments in mice.

1946: The National Multiple Sclerosis Society was formed, and major research grants led to worldwide studies on MS.

1960: The immune system, specifically white blood cells, are implicated in the attack on myelin with MS

1970: The concept of using synthetic myelin to "fool" the immune system into stopping the attacks was born. This led to the development of Copaxone later.

1980s: The CT scan was refined and used to develop a new method of imaging known as MRI, in order to image the brain with MS.

1990: Genetics and MS were further studied, leading to a study of a genetic predisposition.

1993: Betaseron, the first interferon drug was introduced, followed by Avonex and Rebif, and Copaxone. We now had multiple treatments for MS.

2014: We now have 12 disease modifying drugs for MS, and many more on the way!

(Source of Historical Information: National MS Society, 2015.)

For 155 years, since the disease was first described by modern medicine, there were no treatments available at all. In two decades, from 1993-2013, MS went from an untreatable illness to one that can be managed more successfully with 12 disease modifying medications, several being oral drugs instead of injections. Hope is growing, advances are being made daily, and newly diagnosed MS patients today have more promise for a normal life than ever before. We are still waiting for the ultimate cure, but we should take a moment to appreciate how far we have come, how much progress has been made, and how much more awaits us. MS has gone from being shameful and secretive, to something we can openly discuss in support groups, both online and in person.

The internet has made accurate information and support more available and more easily accessible to *every MS patient,* regardless of ability to pay. Drug assistance programs made available by all major drug manufacturers have given every patient the opportunity to be treated. When my grandmother was diagnosed with MS in the 1950s, she was told to "get in bed and stay there." We now know that this is the worst possible advice, and that physical activity is key to remaining healthy with MS. We now recognize that emotional changes are common with MS, and we can seek help for these conditions without shame.

MS patients are undergoing a revolutionary change in the way we cope with this illness. In the past, the disease was shameful and embarrassing to discuss. The social expectation was that you kept your "dirty laundry" to yourself, and you certainly didn't discuss your problems publicly.

Going back to the 1950s when my grandmother had MS, we can clearly see that women in particular were expected to always look and behave in a perfect, feminine way. Women were told to dress a certain way, always act like a "lady," and certainly never complain about your children, your husband, your home, or any family issues. When family members became ill, it was not discussed. When teenage girls got pregnant out of wedlock, they were sent to homes for unwed mothers, birthed babies in secret areas of local hospitals, and were then ushered back home to act as if nothing ever happened. MS was no different in those days, and it was something to hide, lie about, and be ashamed of.

When my grandmother experienced psychiatric symptoms mimicking depression before her MS diagnosis, she was whisked away to a hospital for weeks. At this time, she had several young children at home, but was hospitalized for an extended period of time by her treating physicians. The children were made to interact with her only by writing letters. I have seen these letters, scrawled in the handwriting of a very young child, "I miss you mommy, when will you come home?" I can only imagine the pain this caused my grandparents and their children.

We hear these stories of archaic social attitudes in the 50s and 60s, but we seldom realize that MS was included in these. When I stop to really contemplate this, I realize how fortunate we are to be MS patients in 2015. Look at the changes that have swept over society in the last 60 years. We have seen major changes in minority and women's rights, we have seen freedom and democracy spread worldwide. We are able to speak our minds online without fear of repercussion. No longer do we sit in our homes with curtains drawn and doors closed, hiding our family secret.

We are the generation of MS patients who are exacting real change within the MS community. We are creating beautiful, emotional poems, blogs, and novels about our experience. We are openly sharing the cold, hard facts and the not-so-pretty details of our private experiences with this disease. When I read some of the incredibly gritty, gut-wrenching yet beautiful MS blogs I have found, I am brought to tears. Not only because I can relate so well, but because I was moved by those who were willing to share their most intimate personal and emotional experiences in order to *help others.*

With the power of technology, and our amazing choices of MS related sites, we will never be alone. We should never be made to feel like we need to hide away, in the dark, keeping our secret. We live in a time where honest emotional communication is the new revolution. I encourage you to be a part of that revolution, which is indeed as powerful as any major social change in history.

Never underestimate your power to help other MS patients. Simply by being honest, open, and sharing your life story you can be a healer; and by being honest, we encourage others to be honest and communicate, as well. People are getting *real* and no longer pretending that life is perfect. No one has a perfect life, and now we are reassured to see that others are making the same mistakes, having the same experiences, and going through the same issues as we are.

We have a worldwide audience, and we are each able to reach out to a new generation of patients being diagnosed every day. We should each stop to ask ourselves: "what can I do to share my experience? How can I help another newly diagnosed patient to feel less terrified?" It may be as simple as sharing your story. The power of human connection is one that cannot be overstated, and we are all capable of touching lives simply by sharing openly. The vast expanse of the online community allows us to reach out and touch lives across oceans and continents, without ever leaving our homes. We can benefit from this opportunity, and we can use it to benefit others. We are incredibly fortunate to live in this technological age.

If you begin to lose hope, and you feel that your situation is bleak, try taking a look back at how far we have come. Before 1993, this disease was considered *untreatable.* If we have come this far since 1993, imagine how far we will go in the next 20 years! Research is continuous, and through fundraising efforts, we will find the cure that has been sought since the middle-ages. Have faith, have hope, and stay strong. We have come a long way, don't you agree?

My conclusion is that we need to remember that all human beings are living with unpredictability, and we are not the only ones. The nature of life itself is unpredictable and ever changing, and nothing stays the same, does it? We are in a constant state of change, MS or not. Everything is temporary, for every one of us. We should never spend much time feeling isolated or alone, because when you really think about it, every human being lives with the reality of utter and complete uncertainty.

With chronic illness, especially one like relapsing-remitting MS, reality can change every 15 minutes. We can wake up feeling incredibly great, energetic, rested, and ready for the day. But soon after waking, we may begin to experience weakness, fatigue, and other neurological symptoms. We may begin to experience a full- blown relapse at any moment, even losing the ability to walk, or a sudden visual loss.

This ever-changing reality causes extreme frustration, sadness, and confusion. I found myself with two distinct personalities: My "sick" self, and my "healthy" self. Who would I be today? What if I had plans for lunch with friends? What if I had a twelve-hour work shift scheduled? What if today happened to be Christmas, or another holiday, with dozens of family members coming for dinner? It was incredibly difficult to make *any* plans when life is so unpredictable.

For a period of time, I found myself spending all of my time in my house, unwilling to leave. I was off of work on sick leave after a relapse. I didn't dare make any plans, and I spent my days on the couch, huddled under a blanket. Friends would ask me to meet for coffee or a meal, and I would make up excuses. I was terrified to leave. My mindset had completely changed, and now I thought of myself as damaged, ill, and weak.

I refused to answer my phone, for fear of being asked to meet with friends. I was astounded at how quickly I had changed my entire self-image. I now thought of myself as nothing but sick. The truth was, I was capable of much more than I was doing, but I could not bring myself to get up, get outside, and start to live again.

This is the moment we need to challenge ourselves the most. After we have been knocked down by a relapse, we struggle to get back up. This is the moment we need to use every ounce of strength to regain our lives. If we allow it, MS will completely rule our lives, and this is a dangerous predicament. Beyond the physical challenges of a relapse, we must learn to practice extreme psychological endurance and strength. This is the moment that determines our future: How will we respond *psychologically* to the next relapse? The physical recovery is not entirely within our control, but how about the psychological recovery? This is something we can truly control, and that should make us feel more powerful. The control of our psychological response to relapse is essential to recovery and long-term happiness with MS.

Try to remain in the moment. Get still, quiet, calm, and breathe. Look around at where you really are at this moment. Think of the wonderful, happy things you have in your life and be grateful. Find something to be thankful for, no matter how small. If you are reading these words right now, you are fortunate. There are some who can no longer read the written word. If you understand these written words, be grateful. There are some who don't have the cognitive ability to understand. If you are reading this from a computer, be glad! Most of the world is too impoverished to afford a computer and internet service, or they are kept from reading online posts by a restrictive government.

Don't self-disable. MS is a disabling condition, but we can certainly do far more damage with our own negative inner voices. Maybe you have more ability than you give yourself credit for. Push yourself a bit, and maybe you will be surprised at the abilities you still have right now. It is easy to get into the habit of self-defeating behavior. We might feel that our abilities will not allow us to get up, and try to take a walk. It may be intimidating, and we might be afraid to fall, to look silly in front of other people, or that we might fail. The fear of failure is powerful, and it can prevent you from achieving your goals. Try not to let fear of failure stop you from trying, because you may be closer to success than you ever imagined. That moment that you feel the greatest fear is the moment you must push through anyway.

The key is to start to see your challenges as potential. Anytime you are faced with a *crisis,* a dangerous opportunity, use it to your advantage. With the struggle of MS, we each have the opportunity to become the hero of our own life story. How do you want your life story to be told? You have an opportunity to rise to this challenge, and meet it head on. You may not end up in perfect health, but you may well end up a hero in the eyes of your friends, family, and others struggling with MS.

Journal 14: Hardship, Success, and Memories:

Have you had hardship in your life, MS or otherwise? How have you overcome these challenges? How have you become the hero of your own story? List some techniques for others to learn from, and things you have accomplished despite hardships.

15

Out of the Abyss: Beyond Your Diagnosis

"If you can't fly, then run.
If you can't run, then walk.
If you can't walk, then crawl.
But whatever you do,
You have to keep moving forward."
-Martin Luther King, Jr.

I often watch the news and at times it just depresses me. I am overcome with sadness watching the stories of suffering, deaths of young people, and other violent stories of war and crime. I cannot not imagine going through something as awful as some have. This really got me thinking, though; what are we in for after this life ends? We suffer from a variety of human ailments, cancer, MS, heart disease, and diabetes. We struggle each day to provide food and shelter for our children; we are weak, fatigued, in pain, and trying desperately not to become anxious and depressed. Nothing makes me more upset than hearing stories of young people and children suffering from diseases, hunger, and abuse. Hearing stories of victims of violent crimes, wars, terrorism, and other unexplainable, unjust acts just makes me outraged. Sometimes, life starts to seem like a big waste of time! I often find myself asking: *What is the point of all this?*

I believe in science, evolution, and data. I believe there is a higher power of some sort, and I believe there is some kind of afterlife when this one is over. Would it be the beautiful, light place that we hear about from near death experience survivors? I find great comfort reading books about this topic, including a wonderful book titled *Proof of Heaven,* written by a physician named Dr. Eben Alexander. In this book, Dr. Alexander describes an absolutely stunning, perfect afterlife. In the book, Alexander describes being guided by a "girl with butterfly wings," through a perfect, naturally beautiful world full of love and light. He was sad to leave, wanted to stay, and had no fear of death any longer. Would it be this way? Would it be full of the people we loved who passed before us? Would it be warm, soft, comforting, and perfect?

I certainly hope so. This is where faith comes in, I suppose; this is why faith and religion are so important to human beings. Isn't it difficult to exist with all of this worldly suffering if we don't believe in something greater? I am not traditionally a religious person, but this illness drove me to try to find something to explain all of this. To whom do I issue my complaint if the afterlife is not this perfect place? Who is going to get an earful from me? Who is going to get a piece of my mind if I don't have a mouth to scream with? What if I was just this ethereal, fluid being without any substance? I am going to be angry if this place isn't what we heard it was! I guess my typical response to injustice is always anger; and I get *outraged* if I feel like things are not fair.

Suffering is the ultimate injustice. I hope that everyone who suffered during life and passed away is in a beautiful, peaceful, pain-free place, finally free of the earthly body that caused so much discomfort. So, if I find myself sinking into this angry, outraged place, how did I pull myself out of it, you ask? Here is my answer:

It feels like pulling myself out of a pit of quicksand, slowly climbing up out of the dark place, one arm and one leg at a time, battling a force pulling me down toward the depths; I see the light above, the good things, the happy things, the hopes and dreams. I use every fiber of my being to reach toward that light and climb out of the abyss. I force myself to recall how fortunate I am in so many ways, and how much I have to be grateful for. I try to calm the inner voices and become aware of my surroundings, at peace, and quiet. Some days are more of a struggle than others.

The trick is to force myself to practice the art, (yes I believe it is an art) of gratitude. When your mobility is limited, you may have to scale down the things you can enjoy and be grateful for. However, there are still plenty of things left to experience and treasure. Some ideas:

1. Create love. Surround yourself with people you truly care about, and who support and love you. The more love you give, the more you get. Be the friend you want to have.

2. Enjoy the warmth and light of the sun that shines above you every day. I am always amazed at the mood improvement I experience while sitting in the sun for a while.

3. Take a deep breath and enjoy the feeling of filling your lungs with fresh air.

4. Breathe and enjoy that first smell of rain as it begins to fall. Enjoy the sound of the rain, take in the view of the thousands of prism-like drops as they fall, catching the light in different ways.

5. Look up at the stars above you, and appreciate the vastness of the universe above us.

6. Spend some time with children. There is nothing like the joy and simple pleasures that children experience. A stick, a rock, a piece of paper and pen, a string can become the best thing ever in the eyes of a child.

7. Go out and eat at your favorite restaurant. Enjoy the tastes on your tongue, the sweetness, the salt, the spices. Have a conversation with someone over a meal. Enjoy laughing and recalling mutual experiences, share a dessert!

8. Watch the flames of a warm fire dance in front of you on a cold night. Feel the warmth, watch the oranges and reds and blues move through the flame. Be grateful for the ability to feel these things.

9. Get out of the house and enjoy nature. Crashing waves, singing birds, tall redwood trees, the bloom of desert flowers, the smell of the air when you are out and away from cities.

10. Move your body in whatever way you can. If your legs are weak, move your arms. If your arms are weak, stretch your back. Just move a bit each day. Something is better than nothing.

11. Read and write. Find a book that you love and enjoy it. If you enjoy writing, go for it! Speech technology now allows you to type using only your voice if your hands won't cooperate. If you don't enjoy writing, maybe draw or listen to beautiful music you enjoy.

These are a few of the things I find helpful when being sucked into the void of a depressed mood. If nothing else, these things can distract from the daily experience of MS discomfort. Try it! Maybe even keep a journal of daily gratitude practice. I suppose that none of us will truly know what is in store for us after this life ends. We won't know until that day. Until then, our only option is to have hope, dreams, love, and enjoyment. If we cannot control what happens in the end, at least we can adapt and control how we react to our experiences *today.*

A strikingly meaningful quote I came across:

"You must be shapeless, formless, like water. When you pour water in a cup, it becomes the cup. When you pour water in a bottle, it becomes the bottle. When you pour water in a teapot, it becomes the teapot. Now, water can flow or it can crash. Be water, my friend."
— Bruce Lee

When contemplating your life with MS or any challenge, remember that adaptation is the key to success. Like any living creature must adapt to the environment to survive, we must also learn to change, grow, and learn from our challenges. Every one of us has within the ability to endure, overcome, and in the end, thrive. Take a moment to stop, listen, and appreciate the little things.

I have my "pity party" days. Those days when I believe I have it worse than anyone on Earth. I look around at the rest of the world, the poverty, war, and the suffering. Things could be so much worse, right? Gratitude is a skill, a practice, something you have to work at. I focus on the good things in my life, and do the things I love to do. Find that passion that drives you, and surround yourself with people who are positive and like-minded.

It helps so much to visit MS patient sites, or read MS themed books where you can ask: Has anyone else had a burning sensation on the skin? Has anyone else had a rhythmic buzzing sensation on the legs? Has anyone else had this specific symptom? Even after 5 years with MS, I awake to a new symptom on many mornings. It's like Forrest Gump's "Box of Chocolates." Not only do you "Never know what you're going to get," you hate every single one!

All is temporary, including darkness.

Butterflies are a wonderful example of this. Look at these incredibly beautiful creatures, fluttering and dancing on flowers like living magical fairies from some other world. They live incredibly short lives, but what a beautiful life they lead. These are some of the most graceful, elegant creatures on Earth, but they did not start out this way, did they? These creatures began as rather ugly caterpillars and worms. They become beautiful after a long period of change.

These creatures completely transform every aspect of their lives, and they do it alone. By observing them, we can learn lessons of our own. Their period of change is spent alone, in darkness, with no input from the outside world. They depend on no one during this time, only themselves; and this metamorphosis, or period of transformation, is one of the most miraculous biological phenomena on our planet.

Our period of darkness and transformation begins with our diagnosis of MS. Most of us experience a long period of darkness and crisis from that moment on, lasting for months, or even years. Beginning at the moment of diagnosis, we must completely change our self- image. This is a difficult process, and no one can really help us through it. We must entirely change, and we must do it completely alone.

I often refer to my own years following diagnosis as my "metamorphosis." I changed entirely, and I am not the same person I was before August 24, 2009. Change is difficult, painful, and uncomfortable. Change is awkward, frightening, and exhausting. But, change is an essential part of life. All is temporary, every single thing in this world. This concept helps me get through the tough times, because I am reminded that the darkness will not last forever. All is temporary.

The transition from "healthy" to "MS patient" is not immediate, and we should allow ourselves time to adjust to this new identity. After all, we spent decades of our lives as healthy people before we obtained this new label. How can we adjust to this overnight? When you stop to really ponder it, the diagnosis of an incurable disease truly changes us forever. Not only is it a diagnosis, but a new identity entirely. Accepting a sudden, immediate change in identity is a difficult task. The diagnosis of MS is made on one specific day, and *it is shocking.*

After time, I learned to accept this diagnosis, though it still makes me angry, frustrated, and sad at times. The first year after diagnosis was the most difficult, when my mind struggled to accept. Slowly, though; I began to realize that this was reality. This was part of me, whether I liked it or not. What else was there to do other than accept it? I learned to predict my symptoms more efficiently, to understand which symptoms were familiar and which were new. Acceptance is the final step in the grieving process, and it is defined by the moment you finally begin to feel at peace with your illness. That moment, when you realize that your illness is real, it is manageable, and you have a full life ahead of you regardless.

We each spend a period of time transitioning, accepting, and changing after diagnosis. The most important thing to realize is that it takes time. The way you feel after initial diagnosis; the shock, the anger, the fear, won't last forever. Your life will go on, and it may even be wonderful. MS does not mean that your life is over, rather it means that life has changed. Change is never easy, but it can often lead to great things. Try not to fear the metamorphosis, because you never know how beautiful your life might end up being in the end.

A sense of humor is what gets me through the most difficult days, and it is cheap medicine! Keep your chin up, keep your spirits up, and do your best to tell yourself that things could be worse. Reach out for help if you need it, and find a great MS patient site to access when you need to. Help is out there, and you are most definitely NOT alone!

Remember, you are writing your own life story. Your life is your message to the world, and in the end this is the tale that will be told about you for generations to come. You are slowly, meticulously crafting a brilliant masterpiece that will be the story of *you*. What types of stories do you enjoy reading? Are you drawn to the depressing, dark dramas, or do you find the stories of triumph over tragedy more enthralling? It is fine that you have struggled. Your challenges are part of the story, and they will always be a part of who you are. The key is to make those struggles only a portion of the full story, a piece of the puzzle, not the entire thing. Challenges are opportunities in disguise, for they give you the chance to overcome, succeed, triumph, and win in the end. Those with "easy" lives are not the ones we admire, rather we admire those who have difficult lives, and live them *well*.

Your birth certificate doesn't come with a warranty, much less a guarantee. Your success, happiness, health and longevity are all subject to change without notice. You take possession of your body, as is, no refunds or exchanges. It is recommended that you feed it well and expose it to regular exercise and avoid as many carcinogenic substances as possible. However, even with the best of care, it will ultimately fail. The timing of this event is unknown and unpredictable. The only promise made is that someday it will fail, regardless of your efforts. The sooner we become aware of the fleeting nature of life and understand this, the more likely we are to appreciate the underlying message: That life is a magnificent, transient opportunity. What is infinite, however, is the number of creative, enhancing, uplifting, altruistic, enlightening and loving acts that one may perform while here. *Don't waste a moment.*

Final Journal: Your Story:

Look back at all of the journals you have written. This is YOUR STORY. As they say, life is just a story. Make it a good one. Now, share it with someone you love.

ABOUT THE AUTHOR

Meagan Freeman is a licensed Family Nurse Practitioner who currently resides in Northern California with her husband Wayne and their six children. She is a writer and blogger for several major MS related organizations, including the Multiple Sclerosis Association of America and the Race to Erase MS. Meagan can be found regularly writing her blog *Multiple Sclerosis, Motherhood, and Other Traumatic Experiences.*

Connect Online:

www.motherhoodandmultiplesclerosis.com

Twitter: @MotherhoodandMS